Issues in Clinical Child Psychology

For further volumes:
http://www.springer.com/series/6082

Michael A. Rapoff

Adherence to Pediatric Medical Regimens

Second Edition

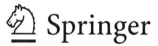 Springer

Michael A. Rapoff
University of Kansas Medical Center
3901 Rainbow Blvd
Kansas City, KS 66160
USA
mrapoff@kumc.edu

ISSN 1574-0471
ISBN 978-1-4419-0569-7   e-ISBN 978-1-4419-0570-3
DOI 10.1007/978-1-4419-0570-3
Springer New York Dordrecht Heidelberg London

Library of Congress Control Number: 2009935393

Printed on acid-free paper

Springer is part of Springer Science+Business Media (www.springer.com)

To my wife, Kim
Who I always love, therefore I always need.

To our children, Lindsey and Nathan and
daughter-in-law Lori
Our hope for the future and the joys of our lives.

To my mother, Shirley Rapoff
For making all of her six children feel special.

In loving memory of my father, Andrew T. Rapoff
Who taught me to be sociable and respect my
elders.

To my siblings, Donna, Danny, Nancy, David,
and Andy
For teaching me to make room for others and lick
the fried chicken legs first.

To Pastor Allen Groff
For showing me that you can love and respect
children.

Preface

Medications don't always work like they should, transplanted organs are rejected, bacteria develop resistance to previously effective antibiotics, and physicians are hampered in their ability to judge the efficacy of treatments they have prescribed. What factors could account for these alarming trends in medicine? One significant factor is that patients and their families don't always adhere to prescribed treatments Haynes, Taylor, & Sackett, 1979. Why this is the case and what can be done about it is the subject of this book.

Before proceeding with this discussion of medical adherence in pediatrics, several caveats are in order:

(1) *It is incumbent on medical providers that they are asking patients to adhere to regimens with demonstrated efficacy.* Providers need to remind themselves of the Hippocratic Oath: "I will follow that system of regimen which, according to my ability and judgment, I consider for the benefit of my patients, and abstain from whatever is deleterious and mischievous" (as cited in Cassell, 1991, p. 145).

(2) *Providers need to abandon the "blame and shame" approach to dealing with medical adherence problems.* It is tempting to blame patients for adherence failures and shame them into changing their behavior. Providers need to share the blame (or better yet omit blame) and look at their own attitudes and behaviors which impact adherence. For example, failing to simplify regimens or minimize negative side effects can adversely impact patient adherence.

(3) *Patients and their families are no longer (or maybe were never) satisfied with a passive role in their health care.* In fact, the term "compliance" lost favor in the literature because it implied for some an authoritarian approach to health care that required unquestioned obedience by patients to provider recommendations (Dimatteo & DiNicola, 1982). Comprehensive and effective health care requires a cooperative relationship between providers and patients and their families. It also acknowledges the following realities, particularly for treating persons with chronic illness:

"Doctors do not treat chronic illnesses. The chronically ill treat themselves with the help of their physicians; the physician is part of the treatment. Patients are in charge of themselves. They determine their food, activity, medications, visits to their doctors – most of the details of their own treatment" (Cassell, 1991, p. 124).

(4) *Finally, children are not little adults.* Pediatric adherence issues are arguably more complex than with adults because of the influences of family members and peers. There are also developmental processes and constraints that uniquely affect adherence for children and adolescents. Caution is in order when extrapolating from theoretical and empirical work with adults and applying this information to pediatric patients.

This volume is intended to give primary and allied health-care providers, researchers, and students an overview of the topic of medical adherence in pediatrics. Chapter 1 reviews definitions of adherence, types of adherence problems, and adherence rates to regimens for acute and chronic diseases. Chapter 2 is a review of the consequences of nonadherence and correlates of adherence. Chapter 3 reviews and critiques adherence theories, such as self-efficacy theory, and the clinical implications of these theories. Chapter 4 describes and critiques different measures of adherence such as assays, electronic monitoring, and self-report measures and also reviews measures of disease and health outcomes. Chapter 5 is a review of educational, organizational, and behavioral strategies for improving adherence. Chapter 6 concludes this book with a summary and critique of adherence intervention studies for acute and chronic pediatric diseases, meta-analyses of pediatric adherence intervention studies, and top ten ways pediatric medical adherence can be improved.

I would like to acknowledge the people who have helped shape the contents of this book and my career in pediatric psychology. I appreciate the feedback and patience of my editor Dr. Michael Roberts as I was way over the page limit with my first draft and insisted on huge tables. I thank my mentor, Dr. Ed Christophersen, for giving me my first opportunities and training in pediatric psychology. I thank my valued physician colleague and collaborator, Dr. Carol Lindsley, for giving me the support and setting for studying ways to help children and adolescents with rheumatic diseases adhere to medical treatments and cope with the demands of a chronic illness. I am grateful to my long-time colleague and friend Dr. Martye Barnard who makes our division run and frees up my time for research and scholarship. I am also very grateful to the patients and families who have participated in our studies and have given me more than I could give them. I appreciate the excellent statistical, research design, and editorial consultations I have received from Dr. John Belmont, Emeritus Professor of Pediatrics. Former students who made significant contributions to our research program on medical adherence include Drs. Carla Berg, Ann Branstetter, Jodi Kamps, and Kathryn Pieper. Two other of my former students who made significant contributions include Drs. Joni Padur and Mark Purviance who are both deceased but are held in loving memory. I am also grateful to the Arthritis Foundation, NIH, and the Bureau of Maternal and Child Health for funding my research on pediatric medical adherence. Finally, a special thanks to my close friend and colleague, Dr. Pat Friman, who helps me avoid piffle in my life and work. Knowing him has helped me to be a better thinker and a better person.

Contents

1 Definitions of Adherence, Types of Adherence Problems, and Adherence Rates 1
Definitions 1
Types of Adherence Problems 3
Adherence Rates to Acute and Chronic Disease Regimens 4
    Adherence to Acute Disease Regimens 4
    Adherence to Chronic Disease Regimens 7

2 Consequences of Nonadherence and Correlates of Adherence 33
Consequences of Nonadherence 33
    Health and Well-Being Effects 33
    Cost-Effectiveness of Medical Care 34
    Clinical Decisions 35
    Clinical Trials 35
Correlates of Adherence to Medical Regimens 36
    Patient/Family Correlates 37
    Disease-Related Correlates 40
    Regimen-Related Correlates 41
    Correlational Cautions and Risk Profile for Nonadherence 42
    Clinical Implications Related to Adherence Correlates 43

3 Adherence Theories: Review, Critique, and Clinical Implications 47
The Health Belief Model 48
    Description 48
    Critical Appraisal 48
    Clinical Implications of the HBM 50
Social Cognitive Theory (Self-Efficacy) 51
    Description 51
    Critical Appraisal 52
    Clinical Implications of SCT (Self-Efficacy) 54

The Theory of Reasoned Action/Planned Behavior   55
  Description   55
  Critical Appraisal   57
  Clinical Implications of the TRA/PB   57
Transtheoretical Model   58
  Description   58
  Critical Appraisal   59
  Clinical Implications of the TTM   61
Applied Behavior Analytic Theory   63
  Description   63
  Critical Appraisal   65
  Clinical Implications of ABA Theory   66
Summary and Implications of Adherence Theories   67

4 **Measurement Issues: Assessing Adherence and Disease
   and Health Outcomes**   69
Why Assess Adherence?   69
  Screening and Diagnosis   69
  Prediction   70
  Intervention Selection   70
  Evaluation of Intervention Efforts   71
What Is to Be Assessed? Selection of Target Behaviors   71
  Guidelines for Selecting Target Regimen Behaviors   71
Who Should Be Assessed and Who Should Assess?   73
How to Assess Adherence? A Critical Review of Assessment Strategies   73
  Drug Assays   74
  Observation   77
  Electronic Monitors   79
  Pill Counts   83
  Provider Estimates   84
  Patient/Parental Reports   86
  Comparative Performance of Adherence Measures   94
Generic Methodological Issues and Recommendations
for Adherence Measurement   102
  Reactivity   102
  Representativeness   102
  Directness   103
  Measurement Standards   103
  Interpretation or What's in a Number?   104
  Clinical and Treatment Utility   105
Assessing Disease and Health Outcomes   106
Methodological Issues and Recommendations for Disease
and Health Measures   108
  Choice of Informants   108
  Representativeness   108

Generic vs. Disease-Specific Measures 109
Psychometric Standards 110
Limiting "Physiogenic Bias" 110
Clinical Feasibility, Utility, and Relevance 111
Conclusions 112

5 Strategies for Improving Adherence to Pediatric Medical
Regimens 115
Educational Strategies for Improving Adherence 116
The "Why?" or Goals of Education 116
The "What?" or Specific Objectives and Content of Education 116
The "How?" of Educational Strategies 117
Summary of Educational Strategies 120
Organizational Strategies for Improving Adherence 121
Increasing Accessibility to Health Care 121
Consumer-Friendly Clinical Settings 121
Increasing Provider Supervision 122
Simplifying and Minimizing Negative Side Effects of Regimens . . . 123
Summary of Organizational Strategies 125
Behavioral Strategies for Improving Adherence 127
Parental Monitoring and Supervision 127
Prompting Adherence 129
Adherence Incentives 129
Discipline Strategies 135
Self-Management Strategies 137
Psychotherapeutic Interventions 138
Summary of Behavioral Strategies 140
Individualizing Interventions: Barriers to Adherence
and Functional Analysis 140
Barriers to Adherence 140
Functional Analysis 141
Technology-Based Interventions 143
Conclusions 145

6 Review of Adherence Intervention Studies and Top Ten
Ways to Advance Research on Adherence to Pediatric
Medical Regimens 147
Intervention Studies on Improving Adherence to Regimens
for Acute Pediatric Diseases 147
Intervention Studies on Improving Adherence to Regimens
for Chronic Pediatric Diseases 151
Meta-Analytic Reviews of Adherence Interventions for Pediatric
Medical Regimens 152

Meta-Analyses of Adherence Interventions for Adults   152
Meta-Analysis of Adherence Interventions for Acute Pediatric
Diseases   177
Meta-Analyses of Adherence Interventions for Chronic
Pediatric Diseases   177
Conclusions from the Meta-Analyses   180
Top Ten Ways to Advance Pediatric Medical Adherence
Research (With Apologies to My Colleagues Who Have Heard
Me Present This at Two Different National Meetings)   181
The Inflated Importance of Adherence   184

References   187
Index   213

Chapter 1
Definitions of Adherence, Types of Adherence Problems, and Adherence Rates

A 10-year-old boy with asthma presents in the emergency room looking pale, having extreme problems breathing and is admitted to the intensive care unit. After several days, his asthma is stabilized and he is sent home. This pattern has been repeated several times over the past several years for this boy. The boy and his mother report that he "usually" takes all his prescribed inhaled and oral medications to treat his asthma and rarely misses a dose. His pulmonary function test results, his frequent visits to the emergency room, and his repeated hospitalizations would suggest otherwise.

Health professionals are all too familiar with the above scenario. There is now over four decades of research documenting that nonadherence to medical regimens is common (around 50% with regimens for chronic diseases) and that it can compromise the health and quality of life of youth with acute or chronic health conditions. This chapter will review how adherence has been defined, the types of adherence problems young people experience, and the studies reporting on adherence rates to regimens for acute and chronic diseases.

Definitions

The term adherence (rather than compliance) has gained acceptance in the literature because it better reflects a more active role for patients and their families in consenting to and following prescribed treatments (Lutfey & Wishner, 1999). Adherence has been defined as "... the extent to which a person's behavior (in terms of taking medications, following diets, or executing lifestyle changes) coincides with medical or health advice" (Haynes, 1979, pp. 1–2). This is the most widely quoted definition in the literature and retains its usefulness because it specifies several important elements related to adherence:

- It brings the focus on specific behaviors which are required of a prescribed medical regimen. Patients are asked to do specific things, such as take medications and follow diets. Specifying behavioral requirements of regimens is a necessary prelude to assessing and improving adherence.

M.A. Rapoff, *Adherence to Pediatric Medical Regimens*, Issues in Clinical Child Psychology, DOI 10.1007/978-1-4419-0570-3_1, © Springer Science+Business Media, LLC 2010

- The word "extent" is an important qualifier related to adherence. It conveys that adherence is not a dichotomous, all-or-nothing phenomenon. There are qualitative and quantitative differences in adherence. For example, nonadherence to medications can take many forms, such as never filling the prescription, omitting doses, doubling up on missed doses, or even overdosing.
- This definition also focuses on the concordance between what patients are being asked to do and what they actually do (if their behavior "coincides" with advice they are given). This implies that there is a standard for judging whether adherence is acceptable or not. This "standard," however, has been rather arbitrary. The oft-quoted standard for adherence – that patients need to take 80% or more of their medications for sufficient treatment effects – appears to have been established based on early research showing that adults who took at least 80% of their medications had their blood pressure drop into the normal range (Dracup & Meleis, 1982). However, this standard has been challenged for diseases such as human immunodeficiency virus (HIV), where patients may need to take 95% or more of antiretroviral medications to control the disease (Osterberg & Blaschke, 2005). More data are needed to develop standards that specify the level of adherence necessary to produce acceptable clinical outcomes for most medical regimens.

A more recent definition has been offered by the World Health Organization, which defines adherence as "the extent to which a person's behavior – taking medication, following a diet, and/or executing lifestyle changes, corresponds with agreed recommendations from a health care provider" (World Health Organization, 2003, pp. 3–4). This definition retains the important elements of the Haynes definition but adds "agreed recommendations," which implies that agreement to follow regimens has been secured from the patient. In pediatrics, this agreement to follow prescribed regimens has to also be obtained from caretakers, particularly for younger children. This definition is also consistent with a more patient-and family-centered approach to adherence that acknowledges that patients and their families make the initial decision to follow a prescribed regimen and to sustain adherence over time. It also places the responsibility on health-care providers to explain treatment options and negotiate with patients and families on what they are willing to do (Adams, Dreyer, Dinakar, & Portnoy, 2004). However, how much health-care providers can negotiate with patients and families without compromising the standard of care is an ethical and potentially legal dilemma. If they compromise care by agreeing to a less-intense regimen and the child has a bad outcome, the health-care provider may open themselves to a lawsuit. Also, while it is clear that adolescents can and should take part in negotiations, there is uncertainty about how much younger children can be involved. Children up to 11 years of age do not always understand the value of preventive medications and find it difficult to understand why someone should take medications when they are not feeling sick (Sanz, 2003). For example, they may not understand why inhaled steroids should be taken to control inflammation for asthma especially when they are not experiencing any breathing problems.

Types of Adherence Problems

There are qualitative as well as quantitative differences in adherence. For medications, families may not even fill a prescription given to them by a health-care provider or they may not refill it in a timely fashion or never refill. Patients may miss or delay doses in a variety of ways. For example, if patients do not take any medications for 3 or more consecutive days, this has been labeled a "drug holiday" (Urquhart & De Klerk, 1998). The possible consequences of taking "drug holidays" is that there is a decline in drug concentrations and actions and if the delay is long enough, the actions can completely fade away. Also, a "rebound effect" can occur once the patient resumes the dosing schedule after a drug holiday resulting in drug toxicities (Urquhart & De Klerk, 1998). Patients may also increase their adherence to medications just a day or two before scheduled clinic visits due to the social desirability effects of wanting to look adherent to the doctor – so-called white-coat compliance. If drug assays are obtained at a clinic visit, it may appear that the patient has been adherent consistently because most drugs have plasma half-lives that are less than 16 h, when in fact the measured plasma level only reflects dosing in the prior 48 h or less, the peak time period for white-coat compliance (Urquhart & De Klerk, 1998). Interestingly enough, the only study that I could find that addressed white-coat compliance in the pediatric literature found no evidence for elevated adherence levels before or after clinic visits for children taking antiepileptic medications (Modi, Morita, & Glauser, 2008). With the advent of electronic monitoring of adherence (see Chapter 4), it is possible to further investigate whether drug holidays or white-coat compliance patterns occur among youth with chronic illnesses.

Another qualitative distinction in the literature is whether nonadherence is unintentional or volitional. Examples of unintentional nonadherence include forgetting to take medications or misunderstanding how to carry out a specific regimen (Adams et al., 2004; Lehane & McCarthy, 2007). It is possible that nonadherence to prescribed regimens may be strategic, rational, and adaptive in certain cases (Deaton, 1985). This type of nonadherence has been described as "volitional," "intentional," "educated," and "adaptive" nonadherence (Adams et al., 2004). The "culture of medical practice" rests on the assumption that patients or their parents seek medical advice and will follow this advice with reasonable fidelity (Vandereycken & Meermann, 1988). Scientifically trained providers find it difficult to understand why people would seek advice, receive empirically validated advice, and then not follow it. Indeed, this does appear to be irrational behavior on the part of patients or their families. But medical treatments sometimes have serious side effects, do not produce anticipated outcomes, or patients find acceptable substitutes. In certain cases, nonadherence becomes rational. One study with adults with HIV found that intentional nonadherence was related to medication side effects. Patients reported that they skipped, altered, or temporarily ceased taking medications because of an adverse drug effect (Heath, Singer, O'Shaughnessy, Montaner, & Hogg, 2002). Other reasons why patients or families may intentionally not adhere are that their treatment goals are different from their provider and the prescribed treatment does not fit into their lifestyle (Adams et al., 2004).

There are, of course, problems with judging whether people intended or did not intend to follow a particular medical regimen. It remains to be seen whether the concepts of unintentional or volitional nonadherence will prove useful in actually designing interventions to address one or the other type of nonadherence. Presumably the distinctions would be helpful. With unintentional nonadherence, we can assist patients who forget doses by providing memory devices (e.g., weekly pill containers, cell phone text messages) to help them remember to take medications. For volitional adherence, we would need to have an honest and open dialog with patients and families to explore the reasons why they would intentionally skip medications or stop taking them and to address their concerns (e.g., reduce negative side effects, competing demands in their daily schedule).

Adherence Rates to Acute and Chronic Disease Regimens

There is wide variability in adherence rates depending on the patient sample and disease, what regimen component is being assessed (e.g., medications, diet, or exercise), how adherence is assessed, and the criteria sometimes used to classify patients as adherent or nonadherent. There is general consensus that nonadherence is higher with regimens for chronic vs. acute diseases. Global estimates are that about one-third of patients fail to finish a course of medications for acute illnesses while adherence averages between 50 and 55% for chronic disease regimens (Rapoff & Barnard, 1991).

Adherence to Acute Disease Regimens

Of the 17 studies reporting on adherence to regimens for acute diseases (see Table 1.1), only one was located since the first edition of this book (Hoppe, Blumenstock, Grotz, Med, & Selbmann, 1999). This new study was a nationwide survey in Germany which examined adherence to medications for acute illnesses in 584 children and adolescents. Similar to previous studies, parents (28.8% of cases) reported their children were adherent, yet the urine assay was negative. There remains considerable variability in adherence rates to medications for acute diseases depending on how and when adherence was assessed (see Table 1.1). Most of the studies reported here used urine assays or pill counts (alone or combined) to assess adherence. Adherence rates varied according to the criterion set by the investigator for classifying patients as nonadherent (or adherent). Take the example of a 10-day course of antibiotics for the treatment of otitis media. In one study, 53% of patients were nonadherent based on the criterion of taking less than half of the prescribed amount (Mattar, Marklein, & Yaffe, 1975). In another study, 5 or 11% of patients (depending on the medication) were nonadherent based on the criterion of taking less than 80% of medications (McLinn, McCarty, Perrotta, Pichichero, & Reindenberg, 1995). Also, these criteria are arbitrary because no biologic basis for determining optimal levels of adherence (in terms of producing acceptable therapeutic effects) has been established for most medical regimens (Gordis, 1979).

Table 1.1 Adherence rates to medications for acute diseases in pediatrics

References	Sample	Disease/regimen	Adherence measure	Results
Bergman and Werner (1963)	N = 59 Mdn age = 2.5 yrs	Pharyngitis or otitis media Penicillin for 10 days	Pill counts Urine assay	>50% stopped taking medications by 3rd day, 71% by the 6th day, and 82% by the 9th day
Charney et al. (1967)	N = 459 Mdn age = 5 yrs	Pharyngitis or otitis media Penicillin for 10 days	Pill counts Urine assay	44% failed to complete the 10-day course; 19% were not taking medication on the 5th day
Daschner and Marget (1975)	N = 105 1.5–13.5 yrs	Recurrent urinary tract infections Antibiotics	Urine assay (twice weekly for 1 week)	29% were "non-takers" and 39% were "irregular"
Dickey, Mattar, and Chudziker (1975)	N = 100 1–12 yrs	Otitis media Penicillin for 10 days	Pill counts Interviews	5% completed the 10-day course; 59% took less than half of the prescribed amount
Disney, Francis, Breese, Green, and Talpey (1979)	N = 75 4–16 yrs	Group A streptococcal pharyngitis Penicillin V or Cefaclor	Urine assay	100% of children had antibiotic present in urine on the 5–8 day of treatment
Feldman, Momy, and Dulberg (1988)	N = 221 (203 evaluated for adherence) M age = 5.1 yrs	Otitis media Amoxicillin or trimethoprim-sulfamethoxazole (10-day course)	Bottle measurement (volume of liquid medication) at home visit	Patients receiving <80% of amoxicillin = 16% and trimethoprim sulfamethoxazole = 8%
Gerber et al. (1986)	N = 195 2–25 yrs	Group A Streptococcal pharyngitis Penicillin V (t.i.d.) or Cefadroxil (q.d.) for 10 days	Urine assay on 9th day of therapy	12% on penicillin 4% on Cefadroxil had negative test for presence of drug
Ginsburg et al. (1926)	N = 198 2–15 yrs	Group A Streptococcal pharyngitis Penicillin V, Penicillin G, Cefadroxil, or erythromycin	Urine assay	6% of children tested negative

Table 1.1 (continued)

References	Sample	Disease/regimen	Adherence measure	Results
Goldstein and Sculerati (1994)	N = 77 0–11 yrs	Otitis media Prophylactic antibiotics	Parent report	23.4% of parents admitted nonadherence
Gordis, Markowitz, and Lilienfeld (1969)	N = 136	Children with history of rheumatic disease Penicillin prophylaxis	Urine assay Interviews	36% children were noncompliers; 32% were intermediate compliers; 32% were compliers
Henness (1982)	N = 198 M age = 7 yrs	Streptococcal pharyngitis Penicillin, erythromycin, or Cefadroxil	Urine assay (5th day of therapy)	6% of children tested negative
Hoppe et al. (1999)	N = 584 0–17 yrs (M = 4.7 yrs)	Tonsillopharyngitis, otitis media, lower respiratory tract infections, or sinusitis Antibiotics	Urine assay Parent report	69.52% had positive urine assay In 168 cases (28.8%), parents claimed regular administration of antibiotic, yet urine test was negative
Mattar et al. (1975)	N = 100 1–12 yrs	Otitis media Antibiotics (10-day course)	Bottle measurement (volume of liquid medication)	59% took less than half of the prescribed medication; only 5% completed the full 10-day course
McLinn et al. (1995)	N = 296 6 mos–8 yrs	Otitis Media Ceftibuten or amoxicillin (10-day course)	Bottle weights	5% of ceftibuten patients and 11% of amoxicillin patients received <80% of medication
Pichichero et al. (1987)	N = 150 4–12 yrs	Streptococcal pharyngitis Cefadroxil or penicillin	Pill count Medication diaries	7 of 145 (5%) patients assessed did not complete the 10-day course
Rabinovich, MacKenzie, Brazeau, and Marks (1973)	N = 118 children (no age range given)	Streptococcal pharyngitis Penicillin G, Penicillin V, or Cephalexin	Urine assay	Of the 74 patients who had an assay, 11% tested negative for presence of drug in urine
Schwartz, Rodriques, and Grundfast (1981)	N = 105 2 mos–17 yrs M = 44 mos	Otitis media Antibiotics (10-day course)	Urine assay (obtained on days 4, 7, and 10 of regimen)	18% had negative tests for two of three assays

Note. Mdn = median; M = mean

Another interesting point about acute disease regimens is that adherence tends to drop over the course of a 10-day regimen (e.g., Bergman & Werner, 1963). This drop makes sense in that children usually start to feel better after the third or fourth day of a 10-day course of antibiotics, which removes a major impetus for adherence (symptom relief) for patients and their parents. It also argues for clinicians to monitor adherence over the course of a regimen to determine when adherence starts to decline and to time adherence interventions to coincide with this decline. Presumably more recent antibiotic regimens that are 5-day courses might produce higher adherence rates, but this remains to be proven.

Adherence to Chronic Disease Regimens

There is also considerable variability in adherence rates for chronic disease regimens depending on the disease, regimen requirements, measure of adherence, and the criteria for classifying patients along adherence dimensions (see Table 1.2). There are 111 studies in Table 1.2 and 78 of them (70%) have been added since the first edition of this book. The new studies are primarily within two newly added disease categories: human immunodeficiency virus (HIV) and gastrointestinal (GI) disorders. One of these new disease categories (GI disorders) represents 23% of the studies in the table, followed by 18% for asthma, and 16% for type 1 diabetes to round out the top three.

The focus of the studies was on adherence to medications in 58% of all studies, on combined regimens (e.g., diet, exercise, and medications) in 19% of them, on diet in 18% of them (primarily gluten-free diet for celiac disease), and on symptom monitoring (blood glucose testing) in 5% of the studies. Encouragingly, 32% of the studies used a more objective measure of adherence, such as electronic monitoring, an assay, or direct observation. Many studies (31%) used a combination of methods to assess adherence, which is recommended because there is no single gold standard for measuring adherence (Quittner, Modi, Lemanek, Ievers-Landis, & Rapoff, 2008).

Several conclusions can be drawn in reviewing the studies in Table 1.2. Adherence rates are higher by parental or youth reports vs. more objective measures of adherence such as assays or electronic monitoring. Also, adherence to regimens tends to drop over time for youth with asthma (Jónasson, Carlsen, & Mowinckel, 2000), cancer (Tebbi et al., 1986), and diabetes (Jacobson et al., 1987; Kovacs, Goldsten, Obrosky, & Iyengar, 1992). Adherence also tends to be higher to medication regimens vs. other non-medication regimens, such as diet or exercise. Of all the disease categories, adherence is relatively higher for medication regimens for HIV/AIDS, which makes sense in that this is a more imminent life-threatening disease. A unique study (Modi et al., 2008) used electronic monitoring of antiepileptic medications for children with seizures and found no evidence for "white-coat compliance" (adherence was not higher before or after clinic visits). Although it is difficult to aggregate adherence rates across or within disease categories, low adherence to medical regimens remains a significant problem, which can threaten the health and well-being of young people with acute and chronic diseases.

Table 1.2 Adherence rates for chronic pediatric disease regimens

References	Sample	Regimen	Adherence measure	Results
Asthma				
Bartlett et al. (2004)	$N = 158$ mothers M age of children $= 7.9$ yrs	Inhaled medications	Mothers' reports	Mothers divided into high and low groups on depressive symptoms "Frequently has problems using inhaler correctly" $= 16.9\%$ of mothers in high group vs. 3.9% in low group "Frequently forgets medicine" $= 22.7\%$ in high group vs. 6.5% in low group "Forgot ≥ 2 days in past 2 weeks" $= 34.8\%$ in high group vs. 16.9% in low group
Bauman et al. (2002)	$N = 1199$ 4–9 yrs ($M = 6.2$ yrs)	Medications and other asthma-control strategies (e.g., buying a mattress cover)	Caregiver report ("Admitted nonadherence" was the number of times caregiver admitted nonadherence with a physician recommendation for asthma management)	"Did not fill a prescription" $= 16.3\%$ "Gives less medicine than prescribed" $= 17.6\%$ "Gives more medicine than prescribed" $= 11.4\%$ "Did not obtain recommended": vaporizer (11.7%), nebulizer (8.8%), dehumidifier (6.9%), peak flow meter (4.8%), air cleaner (4.4%), and mattress cover (3.2%)
Bender, Pedan, and Varasteh (2006)	$N = 5,504$, 5–96 yrs ($n = 423$, 13–20 yrs)	Inhaled steroid/beta agonist combination	Pharmacy refill data	Overall adherence $= 22\%$ of days covered by refills (16% for 13- to 10-year olds)
Berg, Rapoff, Snyder, and Belmont (2007)	$N = 48$ 8–12 yrs	Inhaled steroid	Electronic monitor	Mean adherence $= 69\%$; median $= 71\%$ 65% classified as nonadherent (adherence <80%)

Table 1.2 (continued)

References	Sample	Regimen	Adherence measure	Results
Branstetter, Berg, Rapoff, and Belmont, in press	$N = 60$ 8–12 yrs ($M = 10$ yrs)	Inhaled steroid	Electronic monitor	Mean adherence =66% 40% classified as nonadherent (adherence <80%)
Celano, Geller, Phillips, and Ziman (1998)	$N = 55$ 6–17 yrs	Inhaled steroid	Canister weight	Mean adherence = 44%
Cluss, Epstein, Galvis, Fireman, and Friday (1984)	$N = 22$ 7–12 yrs	Theophylline	Urine assay	50% nonadherent
Coutts, Gibson and Paton (1992)	$N = 14$ 9–16 yrs	Inhaled steroid	Electronic monitor	Underuse recorded on 55% of days and overuse on 2%
Eney and Goldstein (1976)	$N = 43$ 3–16 yrs	Theophylline	Serum assay (therapeutic range = 10–20 μg/ml or higher)	88% of sample had subtherapeutic levels. Median level = 2.65 μg/ml: range=0–15.4)
Jónasson et al. (2000)	$N = 122$ 7–16 yrs	Inhaled steroid Placebo (clinical trial)	Counting remaining doses in inhaler	Adherence lower for adolescents throughout the 27 months of the trial. Adherence to inhaled steroid dropped from 77% at 3 months to 49% at 27 months
Kelloway, Wyatt, and Adlis (1994)	$N = 14$ 12–17 yrs (remainder of sample was 105 patients, 18–65 yrs)	Theophylline Inhaled steroid	Pharmacy claims compared to prescribed orders in medical charts	Theophylline adherence = 73% Inhaled steroid adherence = 30% (both figures lower for adolescents vs. adults)
McQuaid, Kopel, Klein, and Fritz (2003)	$N = 106$ 8–16 yrs	Inhaled steroid	Electronic monitor	Mean adherence = 48%
McQuaid, Walders, Kopel, Fritz, and Klinnert (2005)	$N = 53$ (subsample of $N = 115$) 7–16 yrs	Inhaled steroid	Electronic monitor	Mean adherence = 51%
Miller (1982)	$N = 21$ 12–17 yrs	Theophylline	Serum assay	90% had subtherapeutic levels

Table 1.2 (continued)

References	Sample	Regimen	Adherence measure	Results
Radius et al. (1978)	$N = 80$ 9 mos–17 yrs ($M = 7.7$ yrs)	Theophylline	Serum assay	34% had negative values
Simmons, Gerstner, and Cheang (1997)	$N = 14$ 12–16 yrs	Inhaled beta agonist (salmeterol) vs. placebo (clinical trial)	Electronic monitor	11 of 13 patients (85%) were >85% adherent to salmeterol vs. 7 of 13 (54%) to placebo
Sublett, Pollard, Kadlec, and Karibo (1979)	$N = 50$ 8 mos–14 yrs	Theophylline	Serum assay	98% had subtherapeutic levels, of which 75.5% were due to inadequate adherence and 24.5% were due to physician error (e.g., inadequate doses of medication)
Walders, Kopel, Koins-Mitchell, and McQuaid (2005)	$N = 75$ 8–16 yrs	Inhaled quick-relief (as needed) and longer-term controller (daily) medications	Electronic monitor	Mean daily controller medications taken 46% of time; quick-relief medication use varied between 0 and 251 doses taken over 1 month
Wood, Casey, Kolski, and McCormick (1985)	$N = 111$ 1–20 yrs	Theophylline	Serum assay Caretaker report	34% nonadherent
Zora, Lutz, and Tinkelman (1989)	$N = 17$ 5–13 yrs	Metaproterenol delivered via metered-dose inhaler	Canister weighing Patient/family diaries	2 of 5 children completing 2 weeks of treatment were adherent (40%); 1 of 12 children completing 4 weeks of treatment were adherent (18%)
Cancer				
Festa, Tamaroff, Chasalow, and Lanzkowsky (1992)	$N = 50$ (2 samples with $M =$ 15.6 yrs and $M =$ 19.1 yrs)	Prednisone ($N = 21$) for all Penicillin ($N = 29$) for postsplenectomy prophylaxis	Serum assay for prednisone Urine assay for penicillin	52% nonadherent to prednisone 48% nonadherent to penicillin
Kennard et al. (2004)	$N = 44$ $M = 15.3$ yrs	Trimethoprim/ sulfamethoxazole	Serum assay	27% nonadherent

Table 1.2 (continued)

References	Sample	Regimen	Adherence measure	Results
Lancaster, Lennard, and Lilleyman (1997)	N = 496 5–18 yrs	6-Mercaptopurine	Blood assay	2% had completely undetectable metabolites on one or more occasions
Lansky, Smith, Cairns, and Cairns (1983)	N = 31 2.1–14.3 yrs (M = 7.2 yrs)	Prednisone	Urine assay (<18.7 kgs/cr defined as subtherapeutic)	42% had subtherapeutic levels (M = 19.88; range = 4.95–40.05)
Lau, Matsui, Greenberg, and Koren (1998)	N = 24 2.6–17 yrs	6-Mercaptopurine	Electronic monitor	Mean adherence = 89.4% 33% nonadherent (<90% of doses taken) 17% nonadherent (<80% of doses taken)
Pai, Drotar and Kodish, 2008	N = 51 12–19 yrs	6-Mercaptopurine	Self-report Bioassay	45% reported missing a dose 53% nonadherent by assay
Phipps and DeCuir-Whalley (1990)	N = 54 1 mos–20 yrs (M = 9 yrs)	Antibiotics as part of bone marrow transplant	Review of patient chart and notes from psychosocial team meetings	"Significant" adherence difficulties identified in 52% of sample
Smith, Rosen, Trueworthy, and Lowman (1979)	N = 52 8 mos–17 yrs	Prednisone	Urine assay (<18.7 kgs/cr defined as subtherapeutic)	33% had subtherapeutic levels
Tebbi et al. (1986)	N = 46 2.5–23 yrs (M = 6.85 yrs)	Prednisone	Patient and parent report (corroborated by serum assay). Nonadherence defined as any missed dose during preceding month either "occasional" or "frequent"	Nonadherence rates, postdiagnoses, at 2 wks = 18.8%; at 20 wks = 39.5%; and at 50 wks = 35%

Cystic fibrosis

Table 1.2 (continued)

References	Sample	Regimen	Adherence measure	Results
Czajkowski and koocher (1987)	$N = 40$ 13–23 yrs	Chest physiotherapy, diet, medications, recording daily input and output, and cooperation with medical tests (on inpatient unit)	Medical and nursing notes used to rate degree of adherence (rater not specified)	35% of sample identified as being nonadherent
Hobbs et al. (2003)	$N = 27$ 2–18 yrs	Diet, exercise, chest physiotherapy, inhalation therapy, and medication	Mothers' ratings	Adherence rates to diet (81%), exercise (88%), chest physiotherapy (91%), inhalation therapy (94%), and medication (97%)
Modi et al. (2006)	$N = 37$ 6–13 yrs ($M = 10$ yrs)	Enzymes, airway clearance, nebulized medications, and vitamins	Parent and child report Daily phone diary (DPD) Pharmacy refill (PR) Electronic monitoring (EM)	Mean enzyme adherence = 89.5% by parent report, 90% by child report, 27.4% by DPD, 46.4% by PR, and 42.5% by EM Mean frequency of airway clearance = 74.4% by parent report, 66.9% by child report, and 51.1% by DPD Mean duration of airway clearance = 73.5% by parent report, 69.4% by child report, and 64.2% by DPD Mean combined nebulized medication adherence = 82.4% by parent report, 80% by child report, 47.6% by DPD, and 68.3% by PR Mean vitamin adherence = 88.4% by parent report, 93.8% by child report, 22.2% by DPD, and 33.71% by PR

Table 1.2 (continued)

References	Sample	Regimen	Adherence measure	Results
Passero, Remor, and Salomon (1981)	$N = 58$ (no specific ages given)	Antibiotics, vitamins, chest physiotherapy, and diet	Patient report (nonadherent included partial or poor adherence)	Nonadherence rates for: antibiotics = 7%; vitamins = 10%; chest physiotherapy = 60%; and diet = 71%
Type 1 diabetes				
Anderson, Ho, Brackett, Finkelstein, and Laffel (1997)	$N = 89$ 10–15 yrs	Blood glucose monitoring	Provider rating 3–4 months prior to clinic visit	39% of younger patients (10–12 yrs) monitored blood glucose four or more times daily vs. 10% of older patients ($p < 0.007$)
Hentinen and Kyngas (1992)	$N = 47$ 15–17 yrs	Insulin Diet Glucose monitoring	Patient report (questionnaire) with patient responses used to categorize adherence as high, average, or low	Percent of patients categorized as having high adherence by regimen component: insulin = 72%; diet = 11%; glucose monitoring = 28%
Greening, Stoppelbein, Konishi, Jordan, and Moll (2007)	$N = 111$ 6–16 yrs ($M = 12.30$ yrs)	Blood glucose monitoring, insulin administration, diet, and exercise	Parent report – Self-Care Inventory (SCI), 14 items rated on 5-point Likert scale (1 = "never do it" to 5 = "always do as recommended without fail")	Mean SCI score = 3.85 (SD = 0.66)

Table 1.2 (continued)

References	Sample	Regimen	Adherence measure	Results
Iannotti et al. (2006)	$N = 168$ 10–16 yrs ($M = 13.6$ yrs)	Insulin administration, diet, blood glucose testing, and exercise	Parent and Youth report-modified Diabetes Self-Management Profile, 29 items, structured interview, overall score ranges from 0.00 to 1.00, with higher scores indicating better adherence	Mean score for youth = 0.63 Mean score for parents = 0.65
Jacobson et al. (1987)	$N = 57$ 9–15 yrs ($M = 12.8$ yrs)	Diet Insulin usage Blood glucose monitoring	Health-care provider ratings on a 4-point scale (4 = excellent, 3 = good, 2 = fair, 1 = poor) for each regimen component and a composite index	First 9-month interval mean adherence ratings by regimen: diet = 3.2; insulin usage = 3.3; blood glucose monitoring = 2.8; and composite index = 3 Second 9-month interval mean adherence ratings by regimen: diet = 2.9; insulin usage = 3; blood glucose monitoring = 2.5; and composite index = 2.7 (second 9-month interval significantly lower than first) Adolescents vs. preadolescents had significantly lower adherence to diet, blood glucose monitoring, and the composite index

Table 1.2 (continued)

References	Sample	Regimen	Adherence measure	Results
Jacobson et al. (1990)	N = 61 9–16 yrs	Diet Insulin usage Blood glucose monitoring	Health-care provider ratings on a 4-point scale (4 = excellent, 3 = good, 2 = fair, 1 = poor) Composite index derived from regimen components	Mean adherence ratings by year: Yr 1 = 3.07; Yr 2 = 2.83; Yr 3 = 2.63; and Yr 4 = 2.43
Kovacs et al. (1992)	N = 95 8–13 yrs (M = 11.1 yrs)	Insulin use Glucose monitoring Diet	Diagnosis of medical nonadherence by clinicians based on structured interviews with patients and parents	29.5% of sample were nonadherent Nonadherence emerged an average of 3.5 yrs after disease onset
Lorenz, Christensen, and Pichert (1985)	N = 90 9–15 yrs (M = 12.8 yrs)	Diet	Observations (unobtrusively done in camp setting) Error rate calculated by summing additions and deletions to meal plan divided by the total number of exchanges	Mean error rate = 0.35 (SD = 0.19)

Table 1.2 (continued)

References	Sample	Regimen	Adherence measure	Results
Miller and Drotar (2003)	$N = 82$ 11–17 yrs	Diabetes tasks (e.g., monitoring blood glucose)	Self-Care Inventory ratings of 14 tasks by parents (5-point scale, "never do it" to "always do as recommended without fail") and average number of blood glucose tests over the previous 2 weeks as recorded on glucose meter obtained from medical chart	Mean parent rating = 3.92 and patient rating = 3.93; mean number of glucose tests/day = 2.66
Miller and Drotar (2007)	$N = 63$ 11–17 yrs	Diabetes tasks (e.g., monitoring blood glucose)	Self-Care Inventory ratings of 14 tasks by parents (5-point scale, "never do it" to "always do as recommended without fail") and provider rating of 9 aspects of care. Average number of blood glucose tests over the previous 2 weeks as recorded on glucose meter obtained from medical chart	Mean rating by parent = 3.72 and by provider = 3.25. Mean number of glucose tests/day = 2.77

Table 1.2 (continued)

References	Sample	Regimen	Adherence measure	Results
Naar-King et al. (2006)	$N = 119$ 10–17 yrs	Diet, insulin injections, blood glucose monitoring, and exercise	Ratings by parents and patients (0–100%, assessing "what percent of time do you/your teen" complete each regimen component in past month)	Mean parent rating = 68.04 vs. patient rating = 65.49
Patino, Sanchez, Eidson, and Delamater (2005)	$N = 74$ 11–16 yrs ($M = 13.6$ yrs)	Blood glucose testing, insulin administration, diet, and exercise	Parent and youth report, Self-Care Inventory, 14 items, rated on 5-point Likert scale (1 = "complete nonadherence" to 5 = "complete adherence" over the past month Nonadherence defined as any rating less than complete adherence	Percent of youth who were nonadherent (youth report) to insulin and diet = 49%, blood glucose testing = 75%, and exercise = 64% Percent of youth who were nonadherent (parent report) to insulin and diet = 42%, blood glucose testing = 36%, and exercise = 66%
Schmidt, Klover, Arfken, Delamater, and Hobson (1992)	$N = 69$ 4–18 yrs ($M = 14.2$ yrs)	Diet	Patient dietary records over a 3-day period Registered dietitian tallied the number of food exchanges that deviated from prescribed meal plans	Mean daily deviation from prescribed food exchanges = 23.8% (patients added or deleted, on average, about one of four exchanges)

Table 1.2 (continued)

References	Sample	Regimen	Adherence measure	Results
Stewart et al. (2003)	N = 56 10–23 yrs	Insulin injection, diet, blood glucose testing, exercise, treating reactions, maintaining blood glucose levels, and remembering to do everything every day	Patient rated each care behavior from 20 ("failure") to 100 ("an A+"); average computed across the 7 behaviors to create an adherence composite	Time 1 adherence composite mean = 65.64 vs. time 2 (12–24 months after Time 1) mean = 67.94
Wiebe et al. (2005)	N = 127 10–15 yrs	14 diabetes management tasks	Self-Care Inventory-patient rated adherence to 14 tasks (1 = "never did it" to 5 = "always did as recommended without fail"; average ratings computed across tasks	Mean composite rating = 3.62
Wilson and Endres (1986)	N = 18 12–18 yrs	Blood glucose monitoring	Meters with memory (patients and parents unaware of memory capabilities)	30% of blood tests not performed over 6 weeks. Mean = 40% of blood tests recorded by patient, but not registered by meter. Mean = 18% of blood tests not recorded by patients were registered by meter
Wing et al. (1985)	N = 209 (M = 13.2 yrs)	Blood glucose monitoring	Patient report (frequency of monitoring in the past month)	12% not monitoring 25% monitoring <1X/day 37% monitoring 1–2X/day 26% monitoring ≥3/day

Table 1.2 (continued)

References	Sample	Regimen	Adherence measure	Results
Wing, Koeske, New, Lamparski, and Becker (1986)	$N = 62$ ($M = 13.5$ yrs)	Blood glucose monitoring	Observation of blood glucose monitoring technique by trained observers in clinic	48% estimated blood glucose within 20% of actual value Sterile technique poor; only 10% worked on a tissue or paper towel and none washed hands 40% incorrectly timed test 21% did not adequately wipe blood from testing strip
Gastrointestinal disorders				
Anson, Weizman, and Zeevi (1990)	$N = 43$ 4–19 yrs ($M = 10.7$ yrs)	Gluten-free diet for celiac disease	Classified as adherent or nonadherent by pediatric gastroenterologist based on clinical symptoms and/or signs, histologic findings on a jejunal biopsy specimen, and the presence of antireticulin antibodies in serum	28% classified as nonadherent
Barabino et al. (2002)	$N = 123$ 1–17.2 yrs ($M = 9.8$ yrs)	Azathioprine for inflammatory bowel disease	Health-care provider (person not specified) obtain information on possible causes of treatment discontinuation	3% stopped treatment due to poor adherence

Table 1.2 (continued)

References	Sample	Regimen	Adherence measure	Results
Bazzigaluppi et al. (2006)	N = 143 (M = 8.8 yrs)	Gluten-free diet for celiac disease	Interview by dietician classifying patients as "strict gluten-free diet" = perfect adherence; "occasional gluten intake" = 1–2 episodes of nonadherence per month; "frequent gluten intake" = more than 1 episode of nonadherence a week	39% classified as strict adherence, 46% as occasional nonadherence, and 15% as frequent nonadherence
Cuffari, Théort, and Seidman (1996)	N = 25 9–19 yrs (M = 15.8 yrs)	6-Mercaptopurine for Crohn's disease	Metabolite blood assay	1 patient (4%) nonadherent
Demir et al. (2005)	N = 5 7–14 yrs (M = 9.4 yrs)	Gluten-free diet for celiac disease	Serum anti-gliadin and anti-endomysium antibodies and "clinical condition"	2 patients (40%) had poor adherence
Dohil, Hassall, Wadsworth, and Israel (1998)	N = 4 (M = 12 yrs)	Recombinant human erythropoietin injections for anemia due to Crohn's disease	Patient self-report	1 patient (25%) nonadherent
Ertekin, Selimoğlu, Türkan, and Akçay (2005)	N = 41 2–17 yrs (M = 10.4 yrs)	Gluten-free diet for celiac disease	Serum nitric oxide levels	Data on 23 patients 1 year after gluten-free diet, 4 (17%) were nonadherent

Table 1.2 (continued)

References	Sample	Regimen	Adherence measure	Results
Hartman et al. (2004)	$N = 41$ 5–18 yrs (Mdn = 11 yrs)	Gluten-free diet for celiac disease	"Clinical evaluation" that included interviewing parents and patients plus serum antiendomysial and anti-tissue transglutaminase antibodies	22 patients (54%) nonadherent ("occasional lapses")
Hommel, Davis, and Baldassano (2008)	$N = 36$ 13–17 yrs ($M = 15.69$ yrs)	6-MP/azatinoprine and 5-ASA for Crohn's disease or ulcerative colitis	6-TGN (6-MP metabolite) assay Medical Adherence Measure (MAM): semistructured interview with parents and patients Pill counts	Mean 6-MP adherence: 63% by pill count and 93% by MAM; 81% subtherapeutic by assay Mean 5-ASA adherence: 52% by pill count and 97% by MAM
Kolaček et al. (2004)	$N = 17$ 3–10 yrs ($M = 5.4$ yrs)	Gluten-free diet for celiac disease	Patient report Blood assay (endomysium antibodies) Small bowel biopsy	5 patients (29%) nonadherent by assay and biopsy, but only 4 admitted to lapses
Kumar et al. (1988)	$N = 102$ 12–20 yrs	Gluten-free diet for celiac disease	Patient report	57 patients (56%) reported "strict" adherence, 36 (35%) reported "semi-strict" adherence, and 9 (9%) reported complete nonadherence

Table 1.2 (continued)

References	Sample	Regimen	Adherence measure	Results
Mackner and Crandall (2005)	N = 50 11–17 yrs (M = 14.69 yrs)	Medications for irritable bowel disease	Structured interview with patients and parents who were asked how often medications were taken in the past 2 weeks, with response options 0 = never to 4 = always	Mean child report = 3.37 and parent report = 3.25 (parent and child reports significantly correlated; r = .81, p < 0.001)
Mariani et al. (1998)	N = 47 10–20 yrs (M = 15.2 yrs)	Gluten-free diet for celiac disease	Patient report (3-day diet record) and serologic markers (immunoglobulin antibody assays)	30 patients (64%) reported strict adherence, 14 (30%) admitted lapses once or twice a week, and 3 (6%) admitted consuming a gluten-containing diet. Serologic markers were positive (indicative of nonadherence) for 5 (16%) of the 30 patients reporting strict adherence. Corrected nonadherence rate = 22 of 47 (47%)
Mora et al. (2001)	N = 19 (M = 14.2 yrs)	Gluten-free diet for celiac disease	Serum antibodies	9 patients (47%) nonadherent (positive antibodies)
Murphy, Sood, and Johnson (2002)	N = 44 0.9–14.75 yrs (Mdn = 3.2)	Gluten-free diet for celiac disease	Lactose H_2 breath test before and after starting gluten-free diet (test provides evidence of mucosal healing)	21 patients had positive breath test before starting the diet and 18 of 21 (86%) were positive within 4 weeks and 100% within 8 weeks

Table 1.2 (continued)

References	Sample	Regimen	Adherence measure	Results
Oliva-Hemker, Abadom, Cuffari, and Thompson (2007)	$N = 51$ 5.3–20 yrs ($M = 14.2$ yrs)	Medications (thiopurine immunomodulator and/or mesalamine) for Crohn's disease	Pharmacy refill records (nonadherence defined as <80% of medications dispensed)	50% nonadherent to thiopurine immunomodulator and 66% nonadherent to mesalamine
Ooi, Bohane, Lee, Naidoo, and Day (2007)	$N = 56$ 1.5–17 yrs (Mdn = 12.4 yrs)	Medications (azathioprine or mercaptopurine) for irritable bowel disease	Blood assay of drug metabolites	9 patients (16%) nonadherent
Patwari, Anand, Kapur, and Narayan (2003)	$N = 65$ 2.5–12 yrs ($M = 8.67$ yrs)	Gluten-free diet for celiac disease	Dietary assessment in clinic (not specific how and by whom this was done)	7 patients (11%) classified as "non-compliant/irregular compliance"
Rashid et al. (2005)	$N = 168$ 2–15 yrs ($M = 9.1$ yrs)	Gluten-free diet for celiac disease	Questionnaire completed by patient or parents (with patient involvement)	95% reported strict adherence to the diet
Rodrigues, Johnson, Davies, and Murphy (2007)	$N = 53$ (Mdn = 11.8 yrs) $N = 45$ (Mdn = 12.2 yrs)	Six-week liquid diet therapy (53 on elemental formula and 45 on polymeric formula) for Crohn's disease	Medical records review	72% on elemental formula completed treatment vs. 58% on polymeric formula
Saadah, Zacharin, O'Callaghan, Oliver, and Catto-Smith (2004)	$N = 21$ 1.6–12.9 yrs ($M = 7.5$ yrs)	Gluten-free diet for celiac disease (patients also had type 1 diabetes)	Telephone interview with patient or parent (adherence classified as "excellent," "good," "fair," or "poor"); 20 of 21 interviewed	3 of 20 (15%) classified as fair or poor adherence

Table 1.2 (continued)

References	Sample	Regimen	Adherence measure	Results
Selimoglu, Altinkaynak, Ertekin, and Akcay (2006)	$N = 36$ 2–17 yrs ($M = 10.2$ yrs)	Gluten-free diet for celiac disease	Dietary interview at 6-month follow-up clinic visit (19 children)	2 of 19 (10.5%) not fully adherent to diet
Tommasini et al. (2004)	$N = 30$ 6–12 yrs	Gluten-free diet for celiac disease	Parent report and anti-transglutaminase antibody assay	Parents reported 100% adherence (although admitting "suboptimal compliance on social occasions"); bioassay nonadherence was 28.5% after 18 months (for 8 of 28 patients)
Westman, Ambler, Royle, Peat, and Chan (1999)	$N = 20$ 7.4–17.3 yrs ($M = 12.4$ yrs)	Gluten-free diet for celiac disease (patients also had type 1 diabetes)	Patient report (3-day food record and 7-day food frequency questionnaire)	70% nonadherent to "strict gluten-free diet"
Yachha, Srivastava, Mohindra, Krishnani, and Aggarwal (2007)	$N = 25$ (with "strict adherence" out of 42 enrolled were prospectively studied) 3–14 yrs ($M = 8.3$ yrs)	Gluten-free diet for celiac disease	Serum antiendomysial antibodies	4 of 21 (19%) nonadherent (positive antibody test after 1 year on the diet)
Hiv/aids Dolezal, Mellins, Brackis-Cott, and Abrams (2003)	$N = 48$ Parent/youth dyads 7–14 yrs	Antiretroviral medications	Caregiver and youths' ratings of adherence over past 2 days and previous week	In 46% of caregiver–youth dyads, at least one of the pair reported adherence problems in the last 2 days and 44% reported missing doses in past week; level of agreement among dyads was low (e.g., 38% in disagreement about missed, partial, or off-schedule medications)

Table 1.2 (continued)

References	Sample	Regimen	Adherence measure	Results
Marhefka, Tepper, Farley, Sleasman, and Mellins (2006)	N = 54 2–12 yrs (M = 8 yrs)	Antiretroviral medications	24-h recall interview with caregivers over 3 days "frequency adherence" = % of prescribed doses taken	Mean frequency adherence = 93% 37% missed ≥ 1 dose of medication over 3 days
Martin et al. (2007)	N = 24 8–18 yrs (M = 13.9 yrs)	Antiretroviral medications	Electronic monitor (MEMS) over 6 months (time 1 = average of first 3 months and time 2 = average of last 3 months)	Time 1 mean adherence = 80.9% Time 2 mean adherence = 78.5% Better adherence was significantly associated with lower viral loads and higher CD4 percentages at time 1 and lower viral loads at time 2
Mellins, Brackis-Cott, Dolezal, and Abrams (2004)	N = 75 3–13 yrs (M = 8 yrs)	Antiretroviral medications	Caregiver and youth ratings	40% of caregivers and 56% of children reported missed doses in the past month
Reddington et al. (2000)	N = 90 1.4–14 yrs (Mdn = 7.9 yrs)	Antiretroviral medications	Caregiver ratings of missed doses the day before and last week	15/90 (17%) reported a missed dose the previous day and 39/90 (43%) reported a missed dose in the previous week Nonadherent children had significantly higher viral load (>400 copies/ml) vs. adherent children (50% vs. 24%)
Van Dyke et al. (2002)	N = 125 4 mos–17 yrs	Antiretroviral medications	Caregiver or youth ratings in the past 3 days	70% reported full adherence; 25% reported missing some doses; 5% missed all doses
Williams et al. (2006)	N = 2,088 8–14 yrs	Antiretroviral medications	Caregiver or youth ratings in the past 3 days	84% reported full adherence; lower for 15- to 18-year- olds (76%) vs. younger children (83–89%)

Table 1.2 (continued)

References	Sample	Regimen	Adherence measure	Results
Juvenile rheumatoid arthritis (JRA)				
April, Feldman, Zunzunegui, and Duffy (2008)	$N = 50$ 9–18 yrs ($M = 12.67$	Medications Exercises	Parent and child report, 4 questions per treatment component rated on a 100-mm visual analog scale, with higher scores reflecting higher adherence	Child mean ratings for medications = 84.45 and exercises = 61.60 Parent mean ratings for medications = 83.07 and exercises = 54.88
Brewer, Giannini, Kuzmina, and Alekseev (1986)	$N = 162$ ($M = 9.7$ yrs)	Medications (penicillamine, hydroxychloroquine, or placebo)-drug trial	Pill counts	Patients considered nonadherent if they took <80% of prescribed doses: 14% nonadherent to penicillamine, 12.6% to hydroxychloroquine, and 11% to placebo
Feldman et al. (2007)	$N = 175$ 2–18 yrs	Medications Exercise	Caregiver rated over the past 3 months	Adherence at baseline, 3, 6, 9, and 12 months for medications was 86, 92, 90, 92, and 89%; for exercises 55%, 64%, 61%, 63%, and 54%
Giannini et al. (1990)	$N = 92$ 1.8–15.1 yrs ($M = 7.7$ yrs)	Ibuprofen or aspirin	Pill counts	Patients considered nonadherent if they took <60% of prescribed doses; 3% nonadherent

Table 1.2 (continued)

References	Sample	Regimen	Adherence measure	Results
Hayford and Ross (1988)	$N = 93$ 1.4–20.4 yrs ($M = 8.8$ yrs)	Medications Exercises	Parent and child report – rated how often the child took medications or exercised as prescribed, on a 5-point Likert scale ("never," "seldom," "sometimes," "usually," and "always") Response options always or often defined "positive compliance"	95.1% of parents reported positive compliance with medications vs. 67.2% reporting positive compliance for exercises 89.2% of children reported positive compliance with medications vs. 46.9% reporting positive compliance for exercises For both parent and child report, these differences were statistically significant
Kvien and Reimers (1983)	$N = 25$ 4–15 yrs	Salicylates or naproxen	Pill count	95% adherent overall
Litt and Cuskey (1981)	$N = 82$ ($M = 12$ yrs)	Salicylates	Serum assay (<20 mg/dl defined nonadherence)	45% of patients nonadherent Mean serum level = 21.3 mg/dl
Litt, Cuskey, and Rosenberg (1982)	$N = 38$ ($M = 14$ yrs)	Salicylates	Serum assay (<20 mg/dl defined nonadherence)	45% of patients nonadherent Mean serum level = 20.79 mg/dl
Rapoff, Lindsley, and Christophersen (1985)	$N = 37$ 2–23 yrs ($M = 12$ yrs)	Medications Exercises Splints/wraps	Parent report – asked to rate how easy it was to get their child to take medications, do exercises, or wear splints/wraps (1 = "very hard" to 5 = "very easy")	Means for medications = 4.49; exercises = 3.57; and splints/wraps = 4.33

Table 1.2 (continued)

References	Sample	Regimen	Adherence measure	Results
Rapoff, Belmont, Lindsley, and Olson (2005)	$N = 48$ 2.3–16.7 yrs	Nonsteroidal anti-inflammatory drugs	Electronic monitor	Monitored over 28 consecutive days 48% nonadherent (<80% of doses taken) Median levels showed full adherence on 70% of days, partial on 14%, and no adherence on 7%
Seizures				
Friedman et al. (1986)	$N = 25$ 9–17 yrs	Phenobarbital	Saliva assay (<3.0 μg/ml defined nonadherence)	21% of patients nonadherent Mean saliva level = 5.11 μg/ml
Hazzard, Hutchinson, and Krawiecki (1990)	$N = 35$ 9–16 yrs	Anticonvulsant medications	Serum assay (nonadherence defined as subtherapeutic levels for three separate assays obtained an average of 2.52 months apart)	56% of patients nonadherent
Mitchell, Scheier, and Baker (2000)	$N = 119$ 3.9–13.9 yrs (Mdn = 8.3 yrs)	Anticonvulsant medications	Parent report Serum Assay	Mean adherence by parent report = 88% and by assay = 86%
Modi et al. (2008)	$N = 35$ 2–12 yrs	Antiepileptic drugs	Electronic monitoring (MEMS)	Mean adherence = 79.4% Patients were 100% adherent on 77.1% of days, 50% adherent on 12.7%, and 0% on 10.1% No evidence of "white-coat compliance" (higher adherence before or after clinic visits)

Table 1.2 (continued)

References	Sample	Regimen	Adherence measure	Results
Sickle cell disease				
Barakat, Smith-Whitley, and Ohene-Frempong (2002)	$N = 24$ $M = 7.54$ yrs $N = 73$ primary caregivers	Medications	Nurse ratings (7-point Likert scale, with $1 =$ "not at all adherent" to $7 =$ "extremely adherent") Parent ratings of how often medications taken as prescribed	Mean adherence rating by nurses $= 5.32$ Parents reported medications taken as required, on average, 84.8% of the time
Jensen et al. (2005)	$N = 97$ caregivers Child mean age $= 10.8$ yrs	18 specific regimen requirements, including medications	Caregiver report using the Self-Care Inventory-Sickle Cell (SCI-SC), where parents "rate on a 5-point scale how well their child follows physician advice for 18 specific behaviors" (total scores range from 18 to 90)	Mean SCI-SC total score $= 65$ Individual item mean score $= 4.0$
Olivieri and Vichinksy (1998)	$N = 17$ ($M = 12.3$ yrs)	Hyroxyurea capsules	Electronic monitor (MEMS, n = 10) or diaries (completed by patients or guardians) plus pill counts	4% nonadherent
Transplantation				
Beck et al. (1980)	$N = 21$ 3–20 yrs	Immunosuppressive drug, postrenal transplant	Pill counts	43% of patients were nonadherent (all were adolescents)

Table 1.2 (continued)

References	Sample	Regimen	Adherence measure	Results
Blowey et al. (1997)	$N = 19$ 13–18 yrs	Immunosuppressive drug, post renal transplant	Electronic monitor	21% nonadherent (<80% of doses taken)
Ettenger et al. (1991)	$N = 70$ ($M = 13.5$ yrs)	Immunosuppressive drugs, post renal transplant	Patient report and serum assay	50% nonadherent
Feinstein et al. (2005)	$N = 79$ 1.7–23 yrs	Immunosuppressive drug, post renal transplant	Patient report and plasma assay	16% were nonadherent (all but one of 13 were adolescents)
Gerson, Furth, Neu, and Fivush (2004)	$N = 13$ 2–21 yrs	Immunosuppressive drug, post renal transplant	Electronic monitor and assay	Mean adherence by MEMS = 80% (mean adherence by MEMS for patients classified by assay as probably nonadherent = 69% vs. 95% for those classified as probably adherent)
Kurtin, Landgraf, and Abetz (1994)	$N = 23$ 10–19 yrs ($M = 16$ yrs)	Renal disease Medications Diet	Nurse rated adherence on a 5-point scale ("very often" to "never") Nonadherence defined as those patients rated as "sometimes," "almost never," or "never" adherent	59% of patients rated as nonadherent
Maikranz, Steele, Dreyer, Stratman, and Bovaird (2007)	$N = 70$ 7–18 yrs	Immunosuppressive drug, post liver or renal transplant	Adolescent or caregiver self-report MEMS (electronic monitor)	Mean adherence by self-report = 97% Mean adherence by MEMS = 69%

Table 1.2 (continued)

References	Sample	Regimen	Adherence measure	Results
Penkower et al. (2003)	$N = 22$ 13–18 yrs	Immunosuppressive drug, post renal transplant	Patient report (deemed nonadherent for failing to take medication ≥ 3 times a month)	13.6% nonadherent at baseline and 12 months later
Serrano-Ikkos, Lask, Whitehead, and Eisler (1998)	$N = 53$ Mean age $= 10.2$ yrs	Immunosuppressive drug, post heart or heart-lung transplant	Patient medication diaries and blood assays	70% had good adherence (completed 80% of diaries and blood levels in acceptable range), 21% moderate adherence (unsatisfactory diary completion), and 9% poor adherence (unsatisfactory drug levels)
Shemesh et al. (2004)	$N = 81$ 2–22 yrs	Immunosuppressive drug, post liver transplant	Physicians, nurses, caregivers, and patients ratings ($1 =$ "I always take my medications" to $4 =$ "I rarely take my medications as prescribed") Blood assay	Ratings of 1 ("ideally adherent") were given to 61% of patients by physicians, 52% by nurses, 70% by caregivers, and 70% by patients themselves Only assay levels were significantly correlated with rejection episodes
Tucker et al. (2002)	$N = 68$ (26 African-American and 42 European American) 6–21 yrs	Immunosuppressive drug, post renal transplant	Patient and physician rating, pill counts, and blood assay (all scored on 5-point scale, with $1 =$ "very nonadherent" to $5 =$ "very adherent")	Among African-American patients mean rating by patient $= 3.89$, by physician $= 4.06$, by pill count $= 3.91$, and assay $= 4.13$ Among European American patients, mean rating by patient $= 4.37$, by physician $= 4.02$, by pill count $= 3.58$, and assay $= 4.44$

Chapter 2
Consequences of Nonadherence and Correlates of Adherence

Adherence failures can be costly from a patient's, economic, clinical, and research perspectives. In order to target those patients and families who may need assistance with enhancing their adherence, we need to identify factors which predict adherence. The purpose of this chapter is to review the consequences of nonadherence and studies which have examined predictors of adherence.

Consequences of Nonadherence

Nonadherence to medical regimens can adversely affect the health and well-being of patients, the cost-effectiveness of medical care, clinical decisions, and the results of clinical trials.

Health and Well-Being Effects

Potentially serious health consequences can result from adherence failures. Incomplete adherence to immunosuppressive drugs has been linked to heart, kidney, and liver transplant failures. The 5-year graft survival rate is 72% for living donor kidney transplantations and 60% for deceased donor kidneys for youth between 11 and 17 years old compared to 85 and 77%, respectively, for those between 6 and 10 years. Although the reasons for these lower survival rates in the 11- to 17-year-old group are not fully known, nonadherence with immunosuppressant medications is thought to play a major role (Magee et al., 2004). In one study, about two-thirds of adolescents were found to be nonadherent to immunosuppressant medications, with 15% rejecting their allograft and 26% experiencing graft dysfunction attributed to nonadherence (Ettenger et al., 1991). Another study found a lower 5-year survival rate for kidney transplantation among African-American youth, with nonadherence accounting for 5 out of 7 (71%) graft losses (Jarzembowski et al., 2004). These preventable transplant failures are especially tragic considering the number of children and adolescents who die while waiting for a transplant. Estimates are that approximately 19% of heart, 12% of liver, and 1% of kidney transplant candidates die while

M.A. Rapoff, *Adherence to Pediatric Medical Regimens*, Issues in Clinical Child Psychology, DOI 10.1007/978-1-4419-0570-3_2,
© Springer Science+Business Media, LLC 2010

waiting for a suitable donor (Stuber, 1993). It is also tragic because 1-year survival rates for kidney, liver, and heart transplantation have increased (from 1992 to 2002) to 81–94% (Magee et al., 2004).

Nonadherence has also been implicated in mortality due to asthma in children and adolescents (Sly, 1988). African-American children with asthma are particularly vulnerable, with asthma-related death rates at least five times higher compared to Caucasian children (Goldring, James, & Anderson, 1993; Taylor & Newacheck, 1992). They are also at increased risk for morbidity due to asthma, such as compromised functional status, higher hospitalization rates, and increased school absences (Bauman et al., 2002; Goldring et al., 1993; Taylor & Newacheck, 1992).

Lower adherence to anti-inflammatory medications has been associated with higher active (inflamed) joints for children with juvenile idiopathic arthritis (Feldman et al., 2007). Also, lower adherence to antiretroviral drugs has been associated with higher viral loads in children with HIV/AIDS (Martin et al., 2007; Reddington et al., 2000).

Adherence failures have also been linked to the reemergence of infectious diseases such as tuberculosis (Bloom & Murray, 1992; Gibbons, 1992). These diseases have become more resistant to previously effective antibiotic drugs. Resistance is thought to be caused, in part, by incomplete adherence to medications which exposes offending microbes to less than optimal levels of antimicrobial action, thus making the organism stronger or more resistant to medications. In effect, incomplete adherence can "inoculate" microbial organisms against the effects of medications. This is especially serious given that drug companies are not developing many new types of antimicrobials (Gibbons, 1992). Also, the potential for drug-resistant microbes could be especially threatening to children with compromised immunity, such as those with cancer and cystic fibrosis, who are prone to opportunistic infections.

Adherence failures can also affect the quality of life for patients and their families. For example, children who are nonadherent to their asthma medications can experience more wheezing and variability in their pulmonary function which can limit their daily activities (Bauman et al., 2002; Cluss, Epstein, Galvis, Fireman, & Friday, 1984). Nonadherence has been related to lower quality of life for adolescents who received a liver transplant (Fredericks et al., 2008). Also, nonadherent patients with chronic diseases may be hospitalized or stay home for brief, but repeated periods of time. They then miss school more often, which can adversely impact their academic and social functioning.

Cost-Effectiveness of Medical Care

The cost-effectiveness of medical care can also be reduced by nonadherence (Smith, 1985). Money may be wasted on unused medications or other therapies which are not followed. Nonadherence may also increase unnecessary clinic appointments, emergency room visits, and hospitalizations. The cost of nonadherence in the United

States (including adult and pediatric patients) is estimated to be $100 billion every year (Berg, Dischler, Wagner, Raia, & Palmer-Shevlin, 1993). This includes $8.5 billion just for increased hospital admissions and physician visits (The Task Force for Compliance, 1994). The costs associated with drug-resistant infectious disease are estimated to be between $100 and $200 million a year in the United States alone (Gibbons, 1992). These potentially unnecessary expenses may add to the existing economic burden on families of chronically ill children and society in general, in the form of increased insurance costs and taxes.

There is some evidence that improving adherence can lower the costs of health care, but these studies have been done mainly with adults (Cleemput, Kesteloot, & DeGeest, 2002; Lee, Balu, Cobden, Joshi, & Pashos, 2006). One retrospective study with 137,277 patients (20% of the sample was 18 years or younger) found that higher adherence among patients with diabetes and hypercholesterolemia was associated with lower disease-related medical costs. For those with diabetes, hypertension, hypercholesterolemia, and congestive heart failure, higher adherence was associated with lower hospitalization rates (Sokol, McGuigan, Verbrugge, & Epstein, 2005).

Clinical Decisions

Variations in adherence can also negatively impact medical decisions. If physicians are unaware of adherence problems, they may incorrectly attribute poor outcomes to inadequacies in the treatment regimen and prescribe more potent medicines with more serious side effects. They may also order more invasive and risky procedures to determine the lack of treatment success.

The opposite pattern can also occur. Physicians may overattribute treatment failures to adherence problems, particularly when they use treatment outcome as an indicant for adherence. They may then fail to make appropriate and necessary changes in regimens. For example, medications for adolescents (such as insulin in the treatment of diabetes) need to be adjusted in response to pubertal growth spurts (Barnard, 1986). Without these adjustments, poor treatment outcomes among adolescents may be misattributed to patient nonadherence.

Clinical Trials

Nonadherence can bias clinical trials of promising therapies. Consider an example of a randomized clinical trial comparing a promising new drug (Group A) with a placebo (Group B). Patients are matched on relevant characteristics (age, duration of disease, gender, etc.) and randomly assigned to Group A or Group B. If patients in Group A have less than optimal adherence, then the therapeutic benefits and side effects of the new drug would be underestimated (Urquhart, 1989). Also, a number of studies have shown that patients who adhere to active or placebo medications have better health outcomes compared to poorly adherent patients (Czajkowski, Chesney, & Smith, 2009; Horwitz & Horwitz, 1993). This has been called the "adherence main effect" (Epstein, 1984). Returning to our example, if a comparable number of patients in the placebo group are as adherent as those in the active drug group, there is less likely to be a significant difference in treatment outcomes. Thus, incomplete adherence among patients in the active drug group or adherence main effects would increase sample size requirements for demonstrating a significant difference between the two groups.

Nonadherence can also lead to overestimates of the effectiveness of a newly tested drug. In some trials, investigators discard treatment outcome results for patients who are nonadherent with the test drug or they analyze nonadherent patients' outcome results with the placebo or comparison group (the rationale being they did not really "receive" the new drug). Although, this may be justified when testing a drug under "ideal" circumstances (so-called efficacy trials), it is not acceptable for "effectiveness" trials or the testing of a drug under ordinary circumstances (Fletcher, Fletcher, & Wagner, 1988). Nonadherence can also have a negative impact on pharmacokinetic studies that aim to determine the kinetics of absorption, distribution, and elimination of a drug in the body after administration (Vrijens & Goetghebeur, 1999).

Correlates of Adherence to Medical Regimens

By understanding why patients do or do not adhere to medical regimens, effective interventions can be designed to improve adherence. In turn, this should reduce disease-related morbidity, mortality, and unnecessary health-care costs. In contrast to the adult literature, there are few extant theoretical models which have been proposed and tested that are relevant to pediatric medical adherence (Rapoff, 1996). Most studies have examined correlates or predictors of adherence through correlational/regression analyses or by analyzing between-group differences on variables thought to impact adherence. A few of these types of correlational studies have been based on theoretical models, such as the Health Belief Model (e.g., Bond, Aiken, & Somerville, 1992; Gudas, Koocher, & Wyplj, 1991; Radius et al., 1978). But the vast majority are neither generated by nor linked to any particular theory. This can create a sort of "variance derby" where investigators correlate a myriad of variables to determine which ones account for the most variance in adherence. The result can be no clear "winners" or ostensible winners (e.g., variables such as age and gender), which are spurious or not modifiable.

There are some good reasons for examining correlates of adherence (Rapoff & Christophersen, 1982). *First*, negative correlates of adherence that have been identified consistently can be used to develop "risk profiles" that clinicians can use (with appropriate cautions) to identify patients likely to be nonadherent. *Second*, some adherence correlates that have been consistently related to adherence are modifiable (e.g., complexity of regimens) and therefore can suggest potential remedies (e.g., reducing the complexity of regimens). *Third*, correlates of adherence can be used as matching or control variables in clinical studies. For example, to improve the internal validity of studies, patients can be matched on relevant dimensions (e.g., age, gender, and socioeconomic status) and then randomly assigned to an adherence intervention or control group. *Finally*, correlates of adherence can be used to support or refute existing theories or help generate new theories.

Patient and family, disease, and regimen factors have been most frequently studied as correlates of adherence. The bulk of these studies has examined patient and family correlates of adherence. Each of these types of factors will now be examined, followed by a summary and implications for impacting adherence. Studies that have examined correlates from a specific theoretical position (such as the Health Belief Model) will be reviewed in the next chapter.

Patient/Family Correlates

Demographics. A number of patient- and family-related demographic variables have been associated with adherence. *Adolescents* are more likely to be nonadherent than younger children to regimens for asthma, cancer, cystic fibrosis, diabetes, juvenile rheumatoid arthritis, and to immunosuppressive medications posttransplantation (Anderson, Auslander, Jung, Miller, & Santiago, 1990; Anderson et al., 1997; Beck et al., 1980; Bond et al., 1992; Brownbridge & Fielding, 1994; Feldman et al., 2007; Feinstein et al., 2005; Gudas et al., 1991; Holmes et al., 2006; Jacobson et al., 1987, 1990; Jónasson et al., 2000; Johnson et al., 1992; Kelloway et al., 1994; Kovacs et al., 1992; La Greca, Follansbee, & Skyler, 1990; Patterson, 1985; McQuaid et al., 2003; Serrano-Ikkos et al., 1998; Smith et al., 1979; Stewart et al., 2003; Tebbi et al., 1986; Walders et al., 2005). However, one study found no significant differences in adherence to medications between adolescents and children with juvenile rheumatoid arthritis (Litt & Cuskey, 1981).

A few studies have examined patient *gender* as a correlate of adherence. Males have been found to be less adherent than females to regimens for cystic fibrosis and diabetes (Lorenz et al., 1985; Patterson, 1985; Naar-King et al., 2006). In contrast, an equal number of studies found that females were less adherent than males to regimens for diabetes (Johnson, Freund, Silverstein, Hansen, & Malone, 1990; Patino et al., 2005; Stewart et al., 2003).

Socioeconomic status (SES) and *family composition* variables have also been studied. Lower SES, in general, and lower parental education levels, specifically, have been associated with nonadherence to regimens for asthma, cystic fibrosis, diabetes, juvenile rheumatoid arthritis, and renal disease (Bobrow, Avruskin, & Siller, 1985; Brownbridge & Fielding, 1994; Denson-Lino, Willies-Jacobo, Rosas, O'Connor, & Wilson, 1993; Patterson, 1985; Radius et al., 1978; Rapoff et al., 2005). Parental separation or divorce has been associated with lower adherence to regimens for asthma and renal disease and to immunosuppressive medications after liver, heart, or heart-lung transplantation (Brownbridge & Fielding, 1994; Radius et al., 1978; Serrano-Ikkos et al., 1998; Shemesh et al., 2004). In addition, patients in larger families or where mothers work outside the home are less likely to be adherent to regimens for cancer and cystic fibrosis (Patterson, 1985; Tebbi et al., 1986). One study, however, found that boys with cancer from larger families were more adherent to medications (Lansky et al., 1983).

Race has also been a factor in predicting adherence. Members of minority groups (particularly African-American and Hispanic) have lower adherence to regimens for asthma and seizures (McQuaid et al., 2003; Snodgrass, Vedanarayanan, Parker, Parks, 2001). However, some have argued that entering race into a prediction model is simplistic and not too informative. For example, Tucker and her colleagues have argued for using a "culturally sensitive model," where one studies factors that related to adherence within different racial groups and not between them (Tucker et al., 2001). In some cases, similar factors will be found among racial groups. For example, Tucker et al. (2002) found that difficulty swallowing pills, bad-tasting medications, and complex regimens were associated with lower medication adherence for African-American and European-American children who received a renal transplant (Tucker et al., 2002). In another study, less certainty about when and how to take medications and if medications would keep the transplanted kidney healthy was related to lower adherence among African-American children, while forgetting to take medications was associated with lower adherence among European-American children (Tucker et al., 2001). Existing theories used to generate predictive models may also need to be modified when applied to minority samples. For example, Patino et al. (2005) found no support for Health Belief Model factors (perceived severity and cues to action) in predicting adherence among a sample of primarily African-American children with diabetes.

Knowledge. Patients who are less knowledgeable about their disease and treatment tend to be less adherent to regimens for cancer, cystic fibrosis, and diabetes (Gudas et al., 1991; Holmes et al., 2006; La Greca et al., 1990; Tebbi et al., 1986). In contrast, patient knowledge was not associated with adherence to medications for renal disease (Beck et al., 1980). In one study, older patients had more knowledge about asthma and more responsibility for managing their asthma, but still had lower adherence (McQuaid et al., 2003). A different picture emerges with parental knowledge about their child's disease and treatment. Greater maternal knowledge has been positively related to adherence for preadolescents, but not for adolescents with diabetes and sickle cell disease (Jensen et al., 2005; La Greca et al., 1990).

Patient Adjustment and Coping. Patient adjustment and coping variables have consistently been linked with adherence. On the positive side of the adjustment and coping ledger, higher self-esteem has been associated with better adherence to regimens for diabetes, juvenile rheumatoid arthritis (JRA), and seizure disorders (Friedman et al., 1986; Jacobson et al., 1987; Litt et al., 1982). Greater perceived autonomy and personal independence has been related to higher adherence to regimens for JRA and seizures (Friedman et al., 1986; Litt et al., 1982). Higher social functioning, better disease-specific adjustment, and an internal locus of control have all been associated with higher adherence to diabetes regimens (Jacobson et al., 1987). A sense of optimism has been associated with better adherence to regimens for cystic fibrosis (Gudas et al., 1991) and higher hope has been associated with better adherence to regimens for asthma (Berg et al., 2007). Higher outcome expectancies and self-efficacy have been related to better adherence with regimens for asthma and diabetes (Branstetter et. al., in press; Holmes et al., 2006). Greater problem-solving skills have predicted higher adherence to diabetes regimens (McCaul, Glasgow, & Schafer, 1987).

On the negative side of the adjustment and coping ledger, patients with behavioral or emotional problems are less likely to adhere to regimens for cancer, diabetes, and renal disease (Brownbridge & Fielding, 1994; Greening et al., 2007; Jacobson et al., 1987; Kennard et al., 2004; Kovacs et al., 1992; Miller & Drotar, 2003; Naar-King et al., 2006; Penkower et al., 2003). A history of substance abuse and repeating a grade or dropping out of school has been associated with lower adherence to regimens for HIV and for those receiving liver transplants (Shemesh et al., 2000; Williams et al., 2006). Stressful life events have been associated with lower adherence to regimens for HIV (Williams et al., 2006). The use of "denial" has been related to poorer adherence to cancer medications (Tamaroff, Festa, Adesman, & Walco, 1992) and greater pessimism has been associated with nonadherence to regimens for cystic fibrosis (Gudas et al., 1991).

Family Adjustment and Coping. Turning to the family unit, studies have examined both positive and negative aspects of family and parental adjustment and coping as correlates of adherence. On the positive side, greater family support, expressiveness, harmony, integration, cohesion, and organization have been associated with higher adherence to regimens for cystic fibrosis, diabetes, renal disease, and seizure disorders (Friedman et al., 1986; Hauser et al., 1990; Kurtin et al., 1994; La Greca et al., 1995; McCaul et al., 1987; Patterson, 1985). Also, better communication and problem solving have been associated with higher adherence to regimens for asthma and diabetes (Bobrow et al., 1985; McQuaid et al., 2005). Greater father involvement (in terms of amount and helpfulness) has been related to better adherence for adolescents with asthma, cystic fibrosis, inflammatory bowel disease, phenylketonuria, and spina bifida (Wysocki & Gavin, 2006). Surprisingly, some positive aspects of family and parental functioning have been associated with *lower* adherence to medical regimens. Increased family social and recreational activities outside the home and higher marital satisfaction have been associated with poorer adherence to regimens for cystic fibrosis (Geiss, Hobbs, Hammersley-Maercklein, Kramer, & Henley, 1992; Patterson, 1985).

On the negative side of family adjustment and coping, increased parental stress and poor parental coping have been associated with lower adherence to regimens for JRA and renal disease (Brownbridge & Fielding, 1994; Gerson et al., 2004; Wynn & Eckel, 1986). Poor communication and negative parent–child interactions have been associated with lower adherence to regimens for diabetes and renal disease (Gerson et al., 2004; Lewandowski & Drotar, 2007; Miller & Drotar, 2007). Increased parental depression has been related to poor adherence to regimens for asthma and renal disease (Bartlett et al., 2004; Brownbridge & Fielding, 1994) and greater parental anxiety has been associated with lower adherence to seizure medications (Hazzard et al., 1990). Also, parents who are more likely to place behavioral restrictions on their children tended to have children who were less adherent to their seizure medications (Hazzard et al., 1990). Somewhat surprisingly, parental "nagging" has been associated with better adherence to regimens for diabetes (Burroughs, Pontious, & Santiago, 1993; La Greca et al., 1995).

Parental Involvement/Monitoring. The lack of parental monitoring of treatment-related activities has been found to contribute to nonadherence. Family situations where there is ambiguity about who assumes primary responsibility for regimen tasks or where parental monitoring is low have been associated with lower adherence to regimens for cancer, diabetes, and renal disease (Anderson et al., 1990, 1997; Beck et al., 1980; Bobrow et al., 1985; Feinstein et al., 2005; Holmes et al., 2006; Ingersoll, Orr, Herrold, & Golden, 1986; Tebbi, Richards, Cummings, Zevon, & Mallon, 1988; Wiebe et al., 2005). In one study, parental supervision virtually ceased by the time children with diabetes were 15 years of age (Ingersoll et al., 1986) and in another study, responsibility for taking medication shifted to children who had received a liver transplant when they were 12 years of age (Shemesh et al., 2004). One study found that diabetes-specific, but not general, parental monitoring was associated with higher adherence (Ellis et al., 2007).

Reported Barriers. Patients and their parents are often interviewed or asked to complete questionnaires that assess barriers to treatment adherence. Simply forgetting to take medications is one of the most common barriers reported by patients with asthma and cystic fibrosis and those who received a liver or kidney transplant or their parents (Celano et al., 1998; Modi & Quittner, 2006a; Shemesh et al., 2004; Tucker et al., 2001; van Es et al., 1998). Some patients with asthma and those who received a kidney transplant report that it is difficult for them to swallow pills (Slack & Brooks, 1995; Tucker et al., 2002).

Disease-Related Correlates

Duration. Diseases of longer duration tend to be associated with lower adherence. This is true even among chronic diseases, as longer disease duration has been associated with poorer adherence to regimens for diabetes, JRA, and renal disease (Bond et al., 1992; Brownbridge & Fielding, 1994; Litt & Cuskey, 1981). Also, adherence deteriorates significantly over time to regimens for diabetes, with nonadherence emerging an average of 3.5 years after disease onset (Jacobson et al., 1990; Kovacs et al., 1992).

Course. Adherence to acute disease regimens decreases over the course of the illness, presumably because children start to feel better after 3 or 4 days on an antibiotic regimen. With chronic diseases, symptoms wax and wane over time and adherence may be particularly difficult to sustain during periods when patients are relatively asymptomatic (Rapoff, 1989). Disease course has not been directly investigated in the literature. Most likely, this is because a longitudinal perspective is needed to assess disease course over time and its covariation with adherence.

Symptoms/Disease Severity. It would be reasonable to assume that patients who have more frequent and severe symptoms and higher disease severity would be more adherent in an effort to improve their plight. This has not always been the case. Greater numbers of health problems and hospitalizations and higher disease severity have been associated with lower adherence to regimens for JRA and renal disease (Feldman et al., 2007; Brownbridge & Fielding, 1994). Also, greater seizure activity has been related to lower adherence to anticonvulsant medications (Hazzard et al., 1990). Because these studies assess adherence and symptoms concurrently rather than longitudinally, it is just as likely that lower adherence produced worsening or increased symptoms.

However, some studies have shown the opposite pattern. Higher disease severity has been related to higher adherence among children with JRA (Rapoff et al., 2005) and hospital admission has been related to higher adherence among children with sickle cell disease (Barakat et al., 2002).

Perceived Severity. Here we are speaking of patient or parental perceptions of severity, which appear to be more useful predictors of adherence than those of providers (Rapoff & Barnard, 1991). There is some evidence that parent and patient perceptions are differentially related to adherence. Maternal perceptions of higher severity have been associated with better adherence to medications for asthma (Radius et al., 1978). In contrast, patient perceptions of higher severity have been related to poorer adherence to chest physiotherapy in the treatment of cystic fibrosis (Gudas et al., 1991).

Regimen-Related Correlates

Type and Complexity. Adherence tends to be lower with more complex regimens, such as chest physiotherapy for cystic fibrosis, dietary regimens for diabetes, and exercise regimens for JRA (April et al., 2008; Feldman et al., 2007; Glasgow, McCaul, & Schafer, 1986; Hayford & Ross, 1988; Passero et al., 1981; Rapoff et al., 1985). Lower adherence has been associated with pill vs. liquid medications and for three times daily vs. two times daily medication regimens for HIV (Van Dyke et al., 2002). Adolescents with asthma report that carrying an inhaler with them outside home was a bother (Slack & Brooks, 1995).

Costs. Treatment costs can be prohibitive for some families. For example, one survey with parents of patients with pediatric rheumatic diseases revealed that of those who had a physician visit and purchase of medication in the prior month, 41% reported difficulty paying physician-related charges and 25% had problems paying for medications (McCormick, Stemmler, & Athreya, 1986). Although this study did not correlate costs with adherence, the assumption is that prohibitive costs would lead to poorer adherence. One study found that lower medication costs were related to higher adherence among children with asthma (Bender et al., 2006). Studies are needed to specifically relate the effect of out-of-pocket expenses on adherence.

Side effects. Intuitively, regimens which produce more negative side effects should be associated with lower adherence. For example, chest physiotherapy for patients with cystic fibrosis helps clear the lungs of excessive mucous but results in paroxysms of coughing and gagging. Surprisingly, few studies have examined this factor. Bad-tasting medications have been related to lower adherence to asthma medications (Celano et al., 1998; Radius et al., 1978; Slack & Brooks, 1995; van Es et al., 1998). In contrast, studies have shown that although children may have taste preferences for different antibiotics, these preferences are not differentially related to adherence (El-Charr, Mardy, Wehlou, & Rubin, 1996; Matsui, Barron, & Rieder, 1996). Adverse side effects, either experienced or anticipated, have been associated with lower adherence to regimens for asthma (Buston & Wood, 2000; Slack & Barnes, 1995).

Efficacy. Patient and parent perceptions (rather than providers') regarding the efficacy of medical treatments are most relevant to adherence. Higher levels of perceived benefits as rated by patients and parents have been associated with better adherence to regimens for asthma and diabetes (Bobrow et al., 1985; Bond et al., 1992; McCaul et al., 1987; Radius et al., 1978). A related issue is the immediacy of benefits, which are often delayed for treatments of chronic diseases. For example, an adequate trial of nonsteroidal anti-inflammatory medications in the treatment of JRA is considered to be at least 8 weeks (Lovell, Giannini, & Brewer, 1984). Conversely, patients report not taking medications for asthma because they believe they are ineffective (Buston & Wood, 2000; van Es et al., 1998).

Correlational Cautions and Risk Profile for Nonadherence

Cautions. Before attempting to develop a risk profile for nonadherence and drawing implications for intervention, an important cautionary note is in order: *correlation does not imply causation.* To establish a causal relationship, a minimum of four conditions are necessary: (1) covariation between variables; (2) temporal precedence of the designated causal variable; (3) the absence of alternative explanations for covariance; and (4) a logical connection between variables (Haynes, 1992). The preceding review of adherence correlates generally demonstrates covariation and, in most cases, a logical connection between variables. However, because of the cross-sectional nature of most studies and the complete absence of experimental manipulation of variables, they cannot address temporal precedence or rule out alternative explanations. They can, however, suggest variables that are modifiable and can be experimentally tested for their effect on adherence.

Nonadherence Risk Profile. This review of adherence correlates suggests the following composite "risk profile" for children and adolescents (particularly with chronic disease) who are likely to be nonadherent to medical regimens. They tend to live in families that are preoccupied with dysfunctional interaction patterns, or, by contrast, with positive social and recreational activities outside the home that consume time, energy, and resources necessary for supervising and managing treatment regimens. Their families are also likely to be larger and in the lower socioeconomic strata, possibly with only one parent living at home.

The parents of at-risk children and adolescents tend to have less education in general and/or to be less informed about their children's illness and treatment. Also, the parents may be preoccupied with their own adjustment and coping problems.

The children and adolescents themselves are also likely to have adjustment and coping problems and may be less knowledgeable about their disease and treatment. They are also likely to have primary responsibility for carrying out regimen tasks with little or no supervision from their parents.

At-risk children and adolescents have also had to cope with their disease and treatment over a protracted period, with fluctuations in disease symptoms. In addition, they may be prescribed regimens that are complex, intrusive, costly, have negative side effects, and are not immediately beneficial.

Clinical Implications Related to Adherence Correlates

Some correlates of adherence are static or immutable. For example, what are the clinical implications for considering socioeconomic status as a risk factor for non-adherence to chronic disease regimens (increase family income)? Fortunately, most adherence correlates are modifiable and suggest ways to improve adherence. Even static correlates may be useful in identifying at-risk patients or other modifiable variables that are "marked" by the static variable. For example, adolescence is a relatively static variable. Parents and providers cannot just "wait out" this developmental period with the hope that patients will be more adherent as they get older. Instead, clinicians can identify other factors associated with being an adolescent that impact adherence (e.g., how parents decrease their monitoring of regimen tasks during this period). The following clinical implications focus on modifiable variables that can be altered to improve adherence.

Patient/Family Correlates. One clear overarching implication is that the family needs to be the focus of interventions to improve adherence (La Greca, 1990). This is consistent with the general trend in pediatric psychology for promoting family-based theories and interventions (Kazak, 1997; Roberts & Wallander, 1992; Stark et al., 2005; Wysocki et al., 2006). Patients and their families may need varying degrees of psychosocial support and assistance, ranging from brief and restricted interventions focused on specific adherence behaviors to more comprehensive therapies for enhancing adjustment and coping.

Educational efforts also need to focus on patients and their families. This focus should also include siblings who can have a significant impact on adherence, particularly older siblings who have caretaking responsibilities for younger children with chronic illnesses. However, increased knowledge about diseases and treatments does not always translate into better adherence (McQuaid et al., 2003). It is not enough to know what to do, you have to do it and on a regular basis.

The need for parental monitoring of regimen tasks is taken for granted for younger children who rely primarily or exclusively on their parents to consistently administer medical treatments. However, adolescents also need monitoring by their parents. One reason why adolescents tend to be at risk for nonadherence may be the lack of parental monitoring. Parents should be cautioned not to assume that their teenager is capable of independently carrying out regimen tasks. They should continue to monitor and assist their teenagers in being consistent in following prescribed regimens. Teenagers and parents should be encouraged to share responsibilities for monitoring and carrying out regimens. We also need to clarify the construct of parental monitoring in order to develop adequate measures of this critical predictor of adherence (Ellis, Templin, Naar-King, & Frey, 2008) and separate the effects of general vs. disease-specific types of parental monitoring (Ellis et al., 2007).

There is a subset of patients with chronic diseases and their parents who have significant emotional and behavioral problems, either comorbid with the child's disease or a consequence of having to cope with the demands of a chronic disease. Either way, these families will be additional therapeutic interventions to address their problems, either concurrently or before addressing adherence issues.

Disease-Related Correlates. Patients and their families are more likely to need assistance from clinicians to address adherence issues after the first few years postdiagnosis. When first diagnosed, patients and families may be sufficiently motivated to be adherent in order to control symptoms and minimize disease impact. However, motivation is likely to decrease over time and during relatively asymptomatic periods. Adherence interventions could thus be timed to coincide with these vulnerable periods.

Because the presence of increased symptoms has been associated with poorer adherence, clinicians should assist patients and families in simultaneously monitoring symptoms and adherence. Then, when adherence-enhancing strategies are introduced, they can be more aware of how adherence impacts symptoms and disease course. Also, if patients and families fail to see improved symptom control in spite of adequate adherence, they can negotiate with their physician about changes that can be made in the regimen to improve symptom control.

Perceptions of disease severity by parents and patients are also critical to adherence and may function differently for parents and patients. For parents, emphasizing the potential negative impact or risks of disease may enhance adherence, as they are better able to cognitively process and utilize this information. This may not be the case for children and adolescents who have less ability to process and use this information. Instead, children and adolescents may seek to avoid risk-framed messages and those who deliver it. Thus, clinicians should exercise caution in the way severity or risk messages are communicated to patients and parents. Perhaps, a good compromise would be to communicate risk messages in a positive way by emphasizing the benefits of doing specific and manageable things to prevent or minimize disease severity or risk.

Regimen-Related Correlates. Implications related to regimen factors are very straightforward. Providers must be careful not to overburden families by prescribing unnecessarily complex and costly regimens. Families with ill children have a finite amount of time, energy, and resources to devote to medical regimens, if they are to maintain some semblance of a "normal" family life (Patterson, 1985). Providers must help rather than contribute to this problem of balancing regimen and other family activities. For example, newer antibiotics can be given once a day for 5 days instead of two to three times daily for 10 days to treat acute illnesses. Also, patients can be prescribed generic medications that are less costly to their families and insurance carriers.

Again, parental and patient perceptions enter into the adherence picture in terms of their judgments about the efficacy of prescribed regimens. If they do not perceive that a medical treatment is helpful, patients and families will not continue to consistently follow a regimen or they may discontinue it entirely. So how can providers influence the perceptions of patients and families? One way is to make sure that the most efficacious treatment has been prescribed. Another way is to provide patients and families clear and concise information about the efficacy of regimens that are specific to their situation. This would include traditional measures of outcome (such as disease signs and symptoms and laboratory parameters) as well as quality of life markers (such as increased participation in daily social and recreational activities). Patients and parents can also be trained to monitor some indices of outcome in order to demonstrate to themselves that their efforts to maintain optimal adherence "pays off" in ways that are meaningful to them.

Chapter 3
Adherence Theories: Review, Critique, and Clinical Implications

A theory is "... a set of general or abstract principles based on experimentally established relationships among events used to explain a phenomenon" (Johnston & Pennypacker, 1993, p. 371).

Clinicians might be tempted to skip over this chapter, in part, because discussions of theories often seem pedantic, argumentative, and devoid of practical applications. So, why should clinicians be concerned about theories which speculate about why children and adolescents do or do not adhere to medical regimens? There are two major reasons why clinicians might consider theories.

First, theorizing is ubiquitous and must serve some useful purpose. As soon as humans become language-able, they begin to ask "why" questions. In a very real way, we are driven to make sense of our world, ourselves, and others around us. All clinicians have at least implicit theories about why people think, feel, and behave as they do. By explicating and critically analyzing their theories, clinicians can clarify how they conceptualize and approach adherence issues. The second reason why clinicians should consider theories is to get them out of their "conceptual ruts" (Wicker, 1985). Examining adherence issues from different perspectives will help clinicians find new ways to assess, analyze, and solve adherence problems.

It is easier to justify why researchers should critically examine theories. Like all scientific theories, those which seek to explain why patients adhere or fail to adhere to medical regimens can impact researchers in at least two ways (Johnston & Pennypacker, 1993; O'Donohue & Krasner, 1995). First, theories influence decisions made in planning and conducting studies including the experimental questions, measures, designs, and data analytic procedures. During a lecture to a group of physics students in Vienna, the philosopher Karl Popper gave them the following instructions: "Take pencil and paper; carefully observe, and write down what you have observed." Naturally the students asked what he wanted them to observe, thus making his point that theories precede observations (Popper, 1963, p. 46). Second, theories affect the way investigators react to their data in terms of interpreting and relating their results to other studies, including the body of literature they chose to relate their findings. Finally, in a practical vein, funding agencies require that investigators present an explicit theoretical framework for their research proposals.

This chapter describes, critically appraises, and draws clinical implications relevant to the major theories in medical adherence research. A final section

M.A. Rapoff, *Adherence to Pediatric Medical Regimens*, Issues in Clinical Child Psychology, DOI 10.1007/978-1-4419-0570-3_3,
© Springer Science+Business Media, LLC 2010

will summarize and integrate implications for adherence enhancement as suggested by these theories. The most common theories referred to in the literature will be examined, including the Health Belief Model, Social Cognitive Theory (especially Self-Efficacy), the Theory of Reasoned Action/Planned Behavior, the Transtheoretical Model, and Applied Behavior Analytic theory. With the exception of the Health Belief Model and Applied Behavior Analytic Theory, most of these theories have been formulated and tested only for adults. Therefore, the following discussion will, by necessity, extrapolate from the adult literature in order to apply these theories to children and adolescents.

The Health Belief Model

Description

The Health Belief Model (HBM) has been one of the most widely used theories in health behavior research over the past five decades (Clark & Houle, 2009; Strecher & Rosenstock, 1997). Originally developed in the early 1950s to understand why people failed to take advantage of preventive health services (such as hypertension screening), the HBM was later extended to adherence to prescribed medical regimens (Janz & Becker, 1984; Rosenstock, 1974).

The HBM posits five major sets of variables that predict or explain adherence: (1) *perceived susceptibility* (including the person's perceived risk of contracting or recontracting a condition or acceptance of an existing condition); (2) *perceived severity* (the person's evaluation of the medical and social consequences of contracting an illness or not receiving treatment); (3) *perceived benefits* (the person's judgment of the perceived benefits of taking a particular health action); (4) *perceived barriers* (the person's perception of impediments to adhere to recommended treatments, including a cost-benefit analysis where the person weighs the pros and cons of taking action); and (5) *cues to action* (internal cues, such as disease symptoms or external cues, such as prompting by others that trigger action). In addition, recent formulations of the HBM have included Bandura's concept of self-efficacy (Strecher & Rosenstock, 1997).

The HBM has been adapted for use with pediatric populations. The Children's Health Belief Model (CHBM) is schematically represented in Fig. 3.1 (Bush & Iannotti, 1990). As can be seen, the CHBM not only includes similar dimensions as the classic HBM (e.g., perceived severity), but also emphasizes the role of caretaker influences on children's health beliefs and actions (e.g., caretaker's perceived benefit of the child taking medicines).

Critical Appraisal

Two comprehensive reviews found "substantial empirical support" for the HBM and concluded that perceived barriers were the most "powerful" predictor of a wide range of health practices (Becker, 1974; Janz & Becker, 1984). There is also

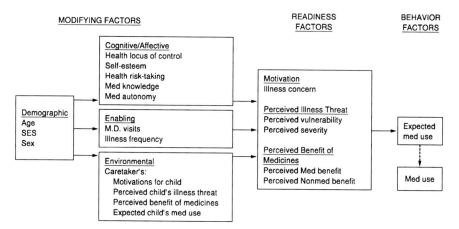

Fig. 3.1 The children's health belief model. Adapted with permission from Bush and Iannotti (1990)

correlational support for components of the HBM in the pediatric medical adherence literature. Higher susceptibility/vulnerability and severity, as rated by mothers, have been associated with better adherence to medications for asthma (Radius et al., 1978) and, as rated by patients, to better adherence to medications for cancer (Tamaroff et al., 1992). In contrast, higher perceived threat or severity, as rated by adolescents, has been associated with lower adherence to regimens for diabetes and cystic fibrosis (Bond et al., 1992; Gudas et al., 1991).

Higher levels of perceived benefits, as assessed by mothers, has been associated with better adherence to asthma medications (Radius et al., 1978) and, as assessed by patients, with diabetes regimens (Bobrow et al., 1985; Bond et al., 1992; McCaul et al., 1987). Consistent with general reviews of the HBM, higher perceived barriers, as rated by parents and adolescents, has been uniformly related to poorer adherence to regimens for asthma and diabetes (Glasgow et al., 1986; McCaul et al., 1987; Radius et al., 1978). The presence of relevant cues to action, as assessed by adolescents, has also been associated with better adherence to diabetes regimens (Bond et al., 1992).

Only one analog study has been conducted with the CHBM (Bush & Iannotti, 1990). This study found that 63% of the variance in children's expected medication use was predicted by the CHBM, with two readiness factors (perceived severity and benefit) accounting for most of the variance. However, this study is limited by its analog nature and failure to measure actual medication use. One study involving primarily African-American youth with diabetes failed to find support for HBM factors in predicting adherence, suggesting that the HBM may not be as relevant for minority populations (Patino et al., 2005).

Despite its track record in the literature, primarily with adults, the HBM can be criticized on the following conceptual and methodological grounds: (1) There are variations in the way HBM constructs have been conceptualized and measured. This has resulted in lack of standardization of measures and variable performance of these constructs as predictors of adherence (Janz & Becker, 1984; Strecher & Rosenstock, 1997). There has been only one measure (The Diabetes Health Beliefs Questionnaire) designed to measure HBM constructs with adolescents who have diabetes and internal reliabilities were sufficient except for the cues to action subscale (Brownlee-Duffeck et al., 1987); (2) Perceptions of health risks (such as perceived vulnerability and severity in the HBM) are subject to an "optimistic bias," or the well-known tendency for people to underestimate their own health risks compared to others (Stroebe & Stroebe, 1995). This may be particularly true of adolescents who tend to view themselves as relatively invulnerable to health risks and behave accordingly by driving too fast, not wearing seat belts, having unprotected sex, and smoking (Coleman & Hendry, 1990; Millstein, Petersen, & Nightingale, 1993); (3) The HBM is limited to accounting for variance in adherence-related behaviors that can be predicted by attitudes and beliefs. Social psychologists have oft cited the tenuous relationship between attitudes and behavior (Stroebe & Stroebe, 1995). Supporters of the HBM acknowledge that changes in health-related behaviors are rarely achieved by direct attempts to change health-related attitudes (Strecher & Rosenstock, 1997). Other influences on adherence need to be considered such as social contingencies, physiologic factors, and perceptions of self-efficacy (Guerin, 1994; Janz & Becker, 1984); and (4) The HBM fails to suggest particular strategies for altering relevant health beliefs. Therefore, there is a dearth of studies designed to experimentally manipulate HBM-related factors to improve adherence (Janz & Becker, 1984). Supporters of the HBM have called for such studies rather than replications of previously confirmed correlational findings (Strecher & Rosenstock, 1997). One promising area in pediatrics is to identify barriers to adherence, which could then presumably be used to tailor interventions to specific barriers for different regimen tasks. Such measures of barriers have been developed for youth with asthma, cystic fibrosis, diabetes, sickle cell disease, and for transplant recipients (Bursch, Schwankovsky, Gilbert, & Zeiger, 1999; Glasgow et al., 1986; Logan, Zelikovsky, Labay, & Spergel, 2003; Modi et al., 2009; Modi & Quittner, 2006a; Simons & Blount, 2007).

Clinical Implications of the HBM

Consider the example of an 8-year-old boy who has moderately persistent asthma that requires daily inhaled anti-inflammatory medication and an inhaled bronchodilator medication as needed. The boy has also been asked to monitor his peak flow levels once per day and after he takes his bronchodilator medication. His parents have been asked not to smoke in the house and to take steps to minimize his exposure to other allergens in the home, such as dust and pet dander. Applying the HBM to this clinical example would suggest the following strategies for assessing and modifying factors related to adherence:

- Perceived susceptibility and severity: The clinician could assess whether the patient and his parents have accepted his condition and have a realistic view of the severity of his asthma. If they have an unrealistic view of severity, the clinician could review peak flow records and encourage the patient and parents to more closely monitor his symptoms in order to gain a more realistic perspective about severity. Information about severity should be balanced with positive information and encouragement that convey a sense of optimism about the patient's and parents' ability to control his disease with increased monitoring and better adherence to prescribed regimens.

- Perceived Benefits: The clinician could assess how confident the patient and parents are that the prescribed regimen is beneficial, especially in terms of quality of life benefits. If confidence is low, the clinician could review potential benefits of the prescribed regimen, such as increased participation in social and recreational activities. Clinicians should be alert to the possibility that prescribed treatments may not be beneficial for particular patients, in spite of optimal adherence. In these instances, the patient and parents should be encouraged to communicate this information to the physician and ask for modifications/additions to increase regimen efficacy.

- Perceived Barriers: The clinician could interview the patient and parents to identify logistic barriers that prevent them from fully adhering to the regimen. For example, taking inhaled bronchodilator medications "as needed" requires the patient or parents to make judgments about "need." They may need assistance in how to monitor symptoms and decide when bronchodilator medications are required. They may need to be instructed to monitor peak flow rates following vigorous exercise and to administer bronchodilator medications if peak flows drop significantly below the patient's baseline levels (see NIH, 1997, for such guidelines). The parents may also perceive multiple barriers to reducing their son's exposure to indoor allergens, such as finding the time to remove dust and pet dander on a regular basis and going outside to smoke. A good general question to ask of patients and parents would be: "What gets in the way or prevents you from doing.....?" The answer to this question should lead to practical recommendations from clinicians (e.g., smoke in the garage).

- Cues to Action: The clinician could assess for the presence of reliable internal and external cues to prompt adherence. If the patient is relatively asymptomatic, there may not be consistent internal cues (such as dyspnea) to prompt adherence behaviors. Therefore, external prompts may be required, such as having the patient set his watch alarm for times when medications are to be taken or encouraging the parents to monitor and prompt adherence behaviors.

Social Cognitive Theory (Self-Efficacy)

Description

Social cognitive theory (SCT) is a comprehensive theory of human behavior originally proposed and promoted by Albert Bandura (1986, 1997). SCT proposes a *triadic reciprocal causation* model that focuses on the interdependence and reciprocal interactions among three major determinants of human agency: behavior, internal personal factors (cognitive, affective, and biological events), and the external environment. The central mechanism of human agency (and the one most relevant to medical adherence) is beliefs of personal efficacy or *perceived self-efficacy*.

Perceived self-efficacy refers to "... beliefs in one's capabilities to organize and execute the courses of action required to produce given attainments" (Bandura, 1997, p. 3). Competent functioning (such as adhering to complex medical regimens) requires both skills and self-beliefs of efficacy to use skills effectively. Children and adolescents who have the necessary skills to perform adherence tasks and a strong belief in their capabilities to perform are more likely to (1) approach difficult regimen tasks as "challenges" to be mastered rather than "threats"; (2) set challenging health-enhancing goals for themselves and remain strongly committed to these goals; (3) increase and sustain efforts to achieve their goals even when they are faced with failure; (4) quickly recover from failures or setbacks to achieve their goals, in part, by attributing these setbacks to knowledge or skill deficiencies, which are remediable; and (5) realize personal accomplishments, reduce stress, and lower their vulnerability to negative affective states, such as depression (Bandura, 1996).

Two major pathways for self-efficacy influences on health have been proposed (O'Leary, 1992). One pathway involves its direct effect on adoption of health practices and adherence to medical regimens. Those high in self-efficacy are more likely to adhere to medical regimens and thereby improve or maintain their health. The other pathway concerns its effect on physiological stress responses. Those high in self-efficacy may experience less stress and negative emotional states, which can exacerbate chronic diseases, such as asthma, arthritis, and diabetes in children and adolescents.

Self-efficacy is thought to be influenced by five major sources (DeVellis & DeVellis, 2001): (1) enactive mastery or learning through experience; (2) vicarious experience or observing competent models; (3) verbal persuasion; (4) physiological states (e.g., viewing physiological arousal as positive energy); and (5) affective states (e.g., positive mood states contribute to a heightened sense of self-efficacy).

SCT also emphasizes the role of *outcome expectancies* or judgments of the likely consequences of one's actions (Bandura, 1997). Self-efficacy judgments (whether one can produce certain actions) are distinguished from outcome expectations (the anticipated consequences of producing actions), but perceived self-efficacy is considered to be the more powerful determinant of behavior (Bandura, 1986). Figure 3.2 is a schematic representation of self-efficacy theory.

Critical Appraisal

SCT and its central construct of self-efficacy has been a robust predictor of human functioning in such diverse areas as cognitive, affective, social, and organizational

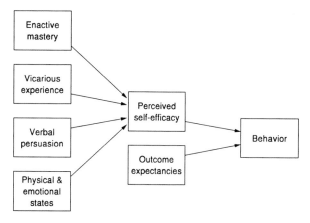

Fig. 3.2 Self-efficacy theory

domains (Bandura, 1997). Self-efficacy has also been an important predictor of a variety of health-related behaviors in adults, including breast cancer screening, smoking, physical exercise, weight control, pain management, and risky sexual behaviors (Bandura, 1997; O'Leary, 1985, 1992; Schwarzer & Fuchs, 1995; Strecher, DeVellis, Becker, & Rosenstock, 1986). Also, the success of self-efficacy as a predictor of health-related behaviors is evident from its more recent inclusion in well-established theories such as the HBM. Although the vast majority of this work has been done with adults, there have been some attempts to develop and validate illness-specific self-efficacy scales for children and adolescents with asthma (Schlösser & Havermans, 1992) and diabetes (Grossman, Brink, & Hauser, 1987). Also, one study found that higher outcome expectancies and self-efficacy among children with asthma predicted greater adherence to inhaled steroid medications (Branstetter et al., in press).

Even the most vocal critics of the self-efficacy theory acknowledge that it is an influential and useful theory in psychology (Catania, 1995; Hawkins, 1995). However, the self-efficacy theory can be criticized on the following conceptual and methodological grounds: (1) Self-efficacy is not a cause, but a reflection of behavior change. It represents an index of the positive and negative outcomes of past performances, a sort of "running average" (Hawkins, 1992). Bandura (1995) counters by citing numerous studies that show self-efficacy retains its predictive power even after controlling for past performance; (2) The self-efficacy theory is also said to minimize environmental influences, including response contingencies and verbally controlled (rule-governed) behavior (Catania, 1995; Hawkins, 1992; Hayes & Wilson, 1995). Bandura has noted that "incentive inducements" or reinforcement contingencies are not sufficient causal agents, particularly as humans gain facility with language and self-referent thought assumes a more critical mediational role in person–environment interactions (Bandura, 1996, 1997); (3) A related criticism is that there is no evidence that self-efficacy (or any other) beliefs have been directly changed. So-called evidence rests on the direct manipulation of some environmental event; no one "randomly assigns" research participants to different levels of self-efficacy (Hayes & Wilson, 1995); and (4) Conceptual confusion has led to variability in how self-efficacy has been operationalized and measured (Corcoran, 1995). Bandura (1996, 1997) acknowledges this criticism and notes that the predictive utility of self-efficacy is attenuated by excessively long intervals between self-efficacy and performance assessments (as self-efficacy may have changed in the interim); the limited scope of self-efficacy assessments (e.g., measuring efficacy beliefs related to dieting, but not exercising when predicting weight loss); global vs. domain-specific assessments of efficacy; and errors in measuring criterion performance variables.

Clinical Implications of SCT (Self-Efficacy)

Consider the example of a 7-year-old female with cystic fibrosis (CF). Her complex and time-consuming medical regimen included the following components: oral pancreatic enzyme replacement to be taken with each meal and snack; increased caloric intake (especially high-protein and high-calorie foods); an inhaled bronchodilator and antibiotic to be taken three times per day; chest physiotherapy three times per day; and DNase (to break up mucus in the lungs) delivered via a nebulizer once a day. This girl also had to take inhaled or oral corticosteroids and intravenous antibiotics, with exacerbations in her disease. She lives in a two-parent family with both parents working outside the home. The patient also has a 6-month-old sister (who does not have CF).

Applying SCT to this clinical example would suggest the following assessment and intervention strategies:

- Although SCT primarily focuses on self-efficacy, it also emphasizes the importance of prerequisite skills for carrying out tasks. The clinician could directly observe how well the patient and parents execute regimen tasks (such as proper technique for using a metered-dose inhaler to deliver bronchodilator and antibiotic medications) and give corrective feedback, training, and practice as needed. This will ensure that the patient and parents know how to carry out regimen components.
- Self-efficacy is the most important and relevant component of SCT. Therefore, the clinician would want to assess self-efficacy perceptions of the patient and the parents. For example, the clinician could ask the parents: "How confident are you in being able to be help your daughter be consistent in taking medications, doing chest physiotherapy, and following dietary recommendations related to CF treatment?" Parents could respond using a five-point scale, ranging from "not at all sure" to "very sure" (Parcel et al., 1994). If parents (or the patient) are not very

confident about managing regimen tasks, efforts can be made to enhance self-efficacy through three major processes: enactive mastery, vicarious experiences, and verbal persuasion (Bandura, 1997).

- Enactive mastery is the most powerful source of self-efficacy and refers to taking steps to ensure that the patient and parents are successful in managing the CF regimen and that they attribute their successes to their efforts. The clinician could provide parents and the patient with social reinforcement for managing regimen tasks and emphasize the importance of their efforts in achieving hard-won successes. Because of the inherent aversiveness of some regimen tasks (such as chest physiotherapy), the patient may need more tangible positive consequences for adherence, such as tokens which can be exchanged for special privileges.
- Vicarious experiences can be promoted by having the patient and parents observe or visualize competent models. For example, the patient and parents could be paired up with other patients and their parents who have encountered and mastered similar problems with regimen tasks.
- Verbal persuasion is the route that most clinicians take to enhance self-efficacy and is most effective if the persuader is viewed as trustworthy and competent. This essentially involves "pep talks" or trying to persuade the patient and parents that they are capable of doing what they need to do. However, clinicians should be careful to avoid overemphasizing this approach and help the patient and parents experience successes in managing the regimen. Otherwise, parents and patients may discount any attempts to boost self-efficacy just by verbal persuasion.
- Clinicians would also need to assess outcome expectancies, particularly patient and parental perceptions of the likelihood that their efforts to manage CF would reap positive benefits. If expectations of beneficial outcomes are low, the clinician may need to emphasize the purpose and potential benefits of prescribed regimens. Also, physicians and nurses can provide disease outcome data (such as pulmonary function test results) or have the patient and parents monitor disease symptoms in order to demonstrate the benefits of prescribed regimens. In some cases, low outcome expectancies are accurate (patients are not benefiting from treatment) and clinicians can refer patients and parents to their medical providers for reassessment of their condition and changes in their regimen.

The Theory of Reasoned Action/Planned Behavior

Description

The Theory of Reasoned Action/Planned Behavior (TRA/PB) is an extension of the Theory of Reasoned Action (TRA) and incorporates predictors from the TRA (Montaño, Kasprzyk, & Taplin, 1997). The TRA was originally introduced in 1967 to help understand why attitudinal measures were often poor predictors of behavior and to improve the predictive utility of attitudinal measures (Ajzen & Fishbein, 1977; Fishbein, 1967). The TRA proposed that attitudinal measures were more

likely to predict behavioral outcomes when measures of both contain four elements:
(1) the *action* or behavior to be performed; (2) the *target* at which the action is
directed; (3) the *context* or situation; and (4) the *time* frame. Thus, attitude–behavior
consistency is more likely if measures of attitudes and behaviors "match" in terms of
the level of specificity across these four elements. The TRA also proposed that the
most proximal determinant of behavior is "intention," or the perceived likelihood of
the person performing the behavior. Behavioral intentions are, in turn, influenced by
a number of factors (see Fig. 3.3).

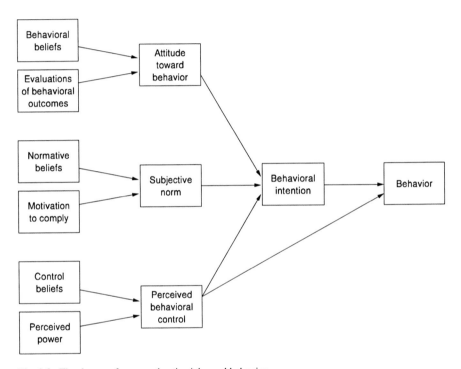

Fig. 3.3   The theory of reasoned action/planned behavior

Intentions are determined by three major factors: (1) *attitude towards the
behavior* (incorporating specific opinions about the behavior and the potential consequences of performing that behavior); (2) *subjective norms* (whether important
people in the person's life approve or disapprove of the action and whether the person is motivated to meet their expectations); and (3) *perceived behavioral control*
(whether the person believes they can perform the behavior and the expected outcome of performing). The construct of perceived behavioral control was the major
variable added to the TRA to form the TRA/PB (Ajzen, 1991). Perceived behavioral
control can influence behavior directly or indirectly through its effect on intentions
(see Fig. 3.3).

Critical Appraisal

The TRA/PB has been applied to the prediction of a variety of behaviors, from academic performance to shoplifting (Clark & Houle, 2009; Stroebe & Stroebe, 1995). These studies tend to provide correlational support for the major components of the theory (Ajzen, 1991). The relatively few studies that have used the TRA/PB to predict health-related behaviors have focused on adults and specific areas such as exercise and mammography screening (Montaño et al., 1997). One study with secondary education students in Holland found that attitudes toward condom use, perceived norms, and perceived control were predictive of intentions to use condoms, while AIDS-related knowledge was not predictive (cited in Stroebe & Stroebe, 1995).

Despite its promise, the TRA/PB can be criticized on several points: (1) Although verbal "intentions" may be useful (particularly when it is hard to measure behavior directly), they are not foolproof (Guerin, 1994). After all, the "road to perdition" is paved by well-meaning intentions. This criticism is particularly relevant when more direct measures of behavior are available and measures of intention are used in place of these direct measures (e.g., asking adolescents with IDDM about their intentions to test blood-glucose levels rather than relying on glucometers that record and store blood-glucose testing results); (2) The degree of specificity of attitudinal and behavioral measures needs to match or be contextually relevant. Mismatches have resulted in low correspondence between attitudinal and behavioral measures; (3) The construct "perceived behavioral control" appears to be conceptually similar to Bandura's construct of self-efficacy (Montaño et al., 1997). This apparent redundancy needs to be evaluated, both conceptually and empirically; and (4) Like all "attitudinal" theories, the burden is on proponents of the TRA/PB to show that experimental manipulations designed to change attitudinal variables actually result in behavior change. However, a meta-analysis of 47 experimental studies of intention–behavior relations (most of which targeted a change in a health-related behavior, such as using sunscreen) did find that a medium-to-large change in intention ($d = 0.66$) led to a small-to-medium change in behavior ($d = 0.36$). The authors concluded that intentions do have a significant impact on behavior but less so than what correlational studies have suggested (Webb & Sheeran, 2006).

Clinical Implications of the TRA/PB

Consider the example of a 15-year-old female with systemic lupus erythematosus (SLE), which is a rheumatic disease that effects multiple organ systems, most notably the musculoskeletal system. The patient's oral medication regimen includes a once-daily antimalarial drug (plaquenil) and a corticosteroid (prednisone) every other day. She also has to avoid exposure to sunlight. The patient lives with her mother and step-father. The patient and her mother have frequent conflicts, which often result in the patient staying over at her friends' house, sometimes during the week and almost exclusively on the weekends.

Applying the TRA/PB to this clinical example might suggest the following strategies:

- Given the centrality of intentions as the most immediate determinant of behavior, the clinician could assess the patient's intentions relevant to her medication regimens. For example, the patient could be asked: "How likely are you to consistently take your medications?" and provided with a three-point response format ("very likely, somewhat likely or not likely"). The clinician could further ask about intentions to adhere to medications at home or when she stays at her friend's home.
- The clinician could also ask about the patient's attitude toward taking the prescribed medications, how significant others (such as friends and parents) react to her regimen (whether they approve or disapprove), whether she believes she is capable of carrying out the regimen, and what she expects to gain by adhering to the regimen.
- If the clinician determines that the patient has weak intentions to adhere to the regimen because significant others provide little support and the patient is doubtful about her ability to be consistent and/or effectively control her disease, then a number of remedial steps can be taken. Perhaps the mother and step-father could provide increased monitoring and support for the patient. In this example, family therapy would be needed to address on-going conflicts so that the mother and step-father could function as agents of support and the patient could be more motivated to meet their expectations.
- In addition (or as an alternative), the patient's friend and her parents could be enlisted as sources of support, since the patient spends many hours at her friend's house.
- To address the issue of low perceived behavioral control, the clinician could ask the patient's physician to provide further information about the purpose and benefits of therapy and disease outcome data that support the efficacy of the prescribed regimen for this particular patient. The patient can also monitor disease symptoms and demonstrate to herself that better disease control occurs when she is more consistent in following her regimen.

Transtheoretical Model

Description

The Transtheoretical Model of Change (TTM) was originally applied to systems of psychotherapy (Prochaska, 1979) and then extended to smoking and other additive behaviors (DiClemente & Prochaska, 1982; Prochaska & DiClemente, 1983; Prochaska, DiClemente, & Norcross, 1992; Prochaska, Johnson, & Lee, 2009).

The TTM has also been recently applied to other health-related behaviors such as exercise, dieting, mammography screening, and diabetes care (Ruggiero, 2000). The TTM focuses on intentional change and has two major dimensions. The first dimension, *stages of change*, specifies "when" shifts occur in attitudinal and behavioral change. In the process of changing a particular health-related behavior (such as quitting smoking), people are said to progress through a series of five stages (Prochaska et al., 2009; Prochaska, Redding, & Evers, 1997): (1) *Precontemplation* (the person has no intention to change in the foreseeable future, usually within the next 6 months); (2) *Contemplation* (the person intends to change within the next 6 months); (3) *Preparation* (the person intends to change in the immediate future, usually within the next month); (4) *Action* (the person has been making overt changes in their lifestyle in the past 6 months); and (5) *Maintenance* (the person is working to sustain changes and avoid relapse). Progression through these stages may not be linear. People may relapse and recycle through previous stages, particularly with addictive behaviors.

The second major dimension of the TTM is *processes of change*, which is concerned with "how" people change. They include overt and covert activities people employ to progress through stages of change (Prochaska et al., 1997).These are empirically supported processes derived from various theoretical perspectives in psychotherapy (thus the term "transtheoretical"). People are said to use different processes at different stages of change. Therefore, interventions designed to help people change should "match" particularly processes to particularly stages of change (see Table 3.1).

Two additional constructs have been added to the TTM (Prochaska et al., 1997). Similar to the HBM and TRA/PB, one construct is *decisional balance*, which refers to a person's relative weighing of the pros and cons of changing. The other construct is *self-efficacy*, adapted from Bandura's self-efficacy theory, but reflecting two components: (1) the degree of confidence people have to cope with high-risk situations without relapsing to unhealthy habits; and (2) temptation or the intensity of the person's urges to engage in an unhealthy habit (e.g., the degree of self-efficacy a teenager has to avoid smoking during a social event with friends who smoke).

Critical Appraisal

The TTM has been applied to a wide range of health-related behaviors with adults, including smoking, weight control, condom use, exercising, and mammography screening (Prochaska et al., 1994, 2009). In general, there has been good empirical support for the major constructs of the TTM (Prochaska et al., 1997). Particular processes of change seem to be employed at different stages of change (e.g., more action-oriented strategies such as reinforcement management employed during action and maintenance stages), consistent with the depiction in Table 3.1. Also, people in the action vs. the contemplation stage tend to discount the costs or cons of changing (Prochaska et al., 1994). The construct of self-efficacy is a

Table 3.1 Stages of change in which particular processes of change are emphasized

Precontemplation	Contemplation	Preparation	Action	Maintenance
Consciousness raising (increasing informationabout self and problem) **Dramatic relief** (experiencing and expressing feelings about one's problems and solutions) **Environmental reevaluation** (assessing how one's problem affects physical environment)	**Self-reevaluation** (assessing how one feels and thinks about oneself with respect to a problem)	**Self-liberation** (choice and commitment to act or belief in ability to change)	**Reinforcement management** (rewarding one's self or being rewarded by others for making changes) **Helping relationships** (being open and trusting about problems with someone who cares) **Counterconditioning** (substituting alternatives for problem behaviors) **Stimulus control** (avoiding or countering stimuli that elicit problem behaviors)	

Note. From "In search of how people change: Applications to addictive behaviors," by Prochaska et al., (1992, pp. 1108–1109). Copyright 1992 by the American Psychological Association. Adapted with permission.

recent and untested addition to the TTM. Given its similarity to Bandura's conceptualization of self-efficacy, it should be a similarly robust predictor of health-related behaviors.

Despite being one of the most popular theories in health psychology, the following conceptual and methodological criticisms can be raised about the TTM (Bandura, 1997): (1) The "stage" aspect of the TTM has been questioned on grounds that human functioning is too complex to be categorized into specific stages. Also, the TTM stages of change violate the three defining properties of a stage theory: qualitative changes across stages (such as Piaget's theory, where preoperational thinking changes qualitatively to operational thinking); an invariant sequence of change (one does not skip stages); and nonreversibility (one does not recycle through stages; for example, an operational thinker does not recycle back to pre-operational thinking, unless a catastrophic event occurs, such as brain damage); (2) It is not clear that change processes are sequenced in the same way across stages for all health-related behaviors. With smoking, people may use cognitive strategies before deciding to quit and behavioral strategies during abstinence. However, for exercise and dietary changes, cognitive and behavioral strategies may increase in tandem across stages (Rosen, 2000); (3) The TTM stages of change are circular in that the stages are defined in terms of the very behavior to be explained. In studies using the TTM, people are categorized into stages based on their self-reports of health-related behaviors, such as smoking and exercising. For example, people might be asked to report how many days per week, how many minutes per session, and how intensely they engage in exercises and whether they intend to increase their exercise activity within the next month (Myers & Roth, 1997). They are then categorized into stages (e.g., in the "precontemplation" stage if they do not exercise and do not plan to in the next month) based on their self-reports of whether they exercise or intend to exercise. This is circular and the correlations between stages and behavior patterns would be spurious; (4) The specific temporal dimension of stages in the TTM appears to be arbitrary and contrived. In studies on addictive behaviors, people have been classified as being in various stages depending on their reported behavior patterns over a 6-month interval (DiClemente et al., 1991) or with exercising, over a 1-month interval (Myers & Roth, 1997). The point here is that one could segment the "stream of behavior" anywhere in time. Also, 6- or 1-month time frames seem ill-conceived when applied to chronic disease regimens. It is difficult to imagine a child recently diagnosed with Type 1 diabetes and her parents "precontemplating" for 6 months about whether insulin should be given to treat hyperglycemia; (5) It remains to be seen whether the TTM is applicable to people with chronic health problems, particularly pediatric populations. TTM developers admit that empirical support for the model comes from studies with convenience or volunteer samples and focus on single, rather than multiple, health-related behaviors (Ruggiero & Prochaska, 1993). Also, the stages and processes which apply to decreasing or eliminating damaging health-related behaviors (such as smoking) are likely to be quite different than those relevant to increasing healthy behaviors (such as exercising); and (6) Although a potential strength of the TTM is the matching of specific behavior change strategies to specific stages of change, there is limited support for the superiority of matched vs. standard or "mismatched" interventions. Also, there is the potential for contradictory recommendations derived from a "transtheoretical" approach that draws from behavioral, psychodynamic, and existential perspectives (Bandura, 1997).

Clinical Implications of the TTM

Consider the example of a 16-year-old male with Type 1 diabetes. His daily regimen is typical of patients with this disease and consists of insulin injections three times per day, blood-glucose testing four times per day, following a meal plan which avoids concentrated sweets, and exercising (while balancing diet and insulin requirements). The patient is active in sports and other extracurricular activities at school and has an active social life. The patient has been diagnosed with diabetes since he was 8 years of age and until recently his disease has been under good control. In the past year, however, control of his disease has been in the "fair to poor" range.

Applying the TTM to this example might suggest the following clinical strategies (Ruggiero & Prochaska, 1993):

- In order to "stage" this patient, the clinician could ask the following questions: "Do you always time your insulin injections, check your blood glucose, follow your special diet, or balance exercising with diet and insulin requirements as you were instructed to do?" The patient would then be classified in one of the TTM stages depending on his choice of one of the following response options for each regimen task: "No, and I don't intend to in the next 6 months" (precontemplation); "No, but I plan to in the next 6 months" (contemplation); "No, but I plan to in the next month" (preparation); "Yes, but for less than 6 months" (action); or "Yes, for more than the past 6 months." (maintenance). Once the patient has been "staged," behavior change strategies suited to his current stage could then be implemented.
- If the patient is in the precontemplation or contemplation stage, the clinician might provide more personalized education, opportunities for emotional expression, and supportive networks. This would allow him to increase his awareness and acceptance of diabetes and increase confidence in his ability to carry out the regimen.
- If the patient is in the preparation stage, the clinician might assist him in setting specific and achievable goals (e.g., testing his blood glucose at least before each meal) and reinforcing any progress (however small) toward meeting these goals. This is a shaping process and the clinician may have to settle for less than optimal performance as long as the patient progresses toward achieving his goals.
- If the patient is in the action stage, the clinician might provide behavioral skills training and self-management strategies, such as self-monitoring and self-reinforcement. Because the patient is trying to establish a new behavioral pattern, he would also require frequent positive reinforcement and social support.
- If the patient is in the maintenance stage, the clinician might help him anticipate and strategize about how to manage obstacles to maintaining adherence. For example, if he goes out to eat with friends, how can he handle social pressures to eat forbidden foods that his friends are eating? Also, the clinician can help the patient cope with lapses in management by putting these into perspective (e.g., "just because I ate the wrong foods today, doesn't mean I have to in the future") and problem solving about ways to cope with future temptations (e.g., "what can I do if I am out with my friends and they are eating what I am not supposed to eat?").

Applied Behavior Analytic Theory

Description

Applied Behavior Analytic (ABA) theory has its historical roots in the foundational work on operant conditioning by B.F. Skinner and has been explicitly related to understanding and modifying adherence to medical regimens (Rapoff, 1996; Zifferblatt, 1975). The ABA model emphasizes two general processes whereby human behavior is shaped: *contingency-shaped* and *rule-governed* behavior (Hayes, 1989; Skinner, 1974).

Contingency-shaped behavior refers to behavior directly shaped by environmental contingencies and its basic form is schematically represented by the *three-term contingency*:

$$S^D \rightarrow R \rightarrow S$$

For example, a discriminative stimulus (pain) sets the occasion for or prompts a response (taking pain medications) and the probability of that response is altered by a consequent stimulus (pain relief).

Four basic operant processes can be distinguished based on whether a consequence is added or subtracted contingent on a behavior and the resulting effect on behavior in terms of increasing or decreasing the probability of that behavior in the future (see Fig. 3.4). *Positive reinforcement* occurs when a response-contingent consequence increases a behavior (e.g., symptom relief increases the probability the person will take prescribed medications). In contrast, *positive punishment* occurs when a response-contingent consequence decreases a behavior (e.g., taking prescribed medications results in negative side effects, thereby "punishing" medication-taking). *Negative reinforcement* occurs when response-contingent removal of a consequence increases a behavior (e.g., taking antacids terminates or allows one to avoid gastrointestinal irritation caused by some medications). *Negative punishment* (or extinction) occurs when response-contingent removal of a consequence decreases a behavior (e.g., a child does not comply with a parental request to take medications and loses privileges).

Behavior analysts are also giving increased attention to the unique role of verbal antecedents in the control of human behavior; so-called, rule-governed behavior (Hayes, 1989). Rules are ubiquitous and can take many forms, such as instructions, laws, maxims, proverbs, advice, grammar, and scientific propositions (Riegler & Baer, 1989). They are valuable because people can learn them more quickly without having directly experienced (or without ever experiencing) the consequences implied or specified by the rule (Skinner, 1974; Riegler & Baer, 1989). Parents count on rules, such as "look both ways before crossing the street," to keep their children out of harms' way

Whether rules are followed or not depends on the following factors (Hayes, 1989; Riegler & Baer, 1989): (1) a generalized history of reinforcement for following rules

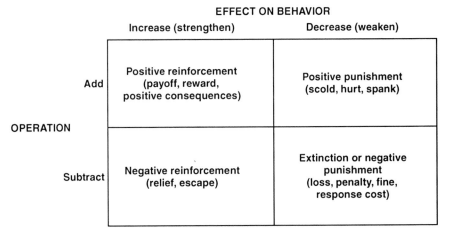

Fig. 3.4 Operant theory

(or punishment for failing to follow rules); (2) immediate local consequences for following rules (often in the form of social approval or disapproval); (3) contact with the contingencies described in a rule (e.g., taking medications and experiencing symptom relief); and (4) automatic or self-given consequences (e.g., positive or negative feelings and thoughts)

There are, however, problems and limitations of rule-governed behavior. Children may not be able to follow rules because they lack the prerequisite skills (Poppen, 1989). Also, following rules may result in negative consequences, such as taking medications and experiencing aversive side effects. Children may also fail to generate rules when it is advantageous to do so or they may form inaccurate or unrealistic rules (Hayes, Kohlenberg, & Melancon, 1989). For example, a teenager with lupus in one of our studies said she took steroid medication more often or less often than prescribed, depending on how she felt (Pieper, Rapoff, Purviance, & Lindsley, 1989). This rule was unhelpful because by following this rule she did adequately control the symptoms of her disease.

A critical dimension of the ABA approach is doing a functional analysis, which involves identifying "... important, controllable, causal functional relationships applicable to a specified set of target behaviors for an individual client" (Haynes & O'Brien, 1990, p. 654). Relating this approach to medical adherence would involve the following steps: (1) operationally defining adherence behaviors; (2) identifying antecedent events that set the occasion for or predict adherence behaviors; (3) generating hypotheses about consequences that maintain adherence behaviors; (4) collecting observational data (when feasible) to provide at least correlational confirmation of the hypothesized associations of antecedent and consequent events with adherence behaviors (Horner, 1994; Yoman, 2008). Once the functional analysis is completed, a treatment plan can be formulated, implemented, and tested.

Critical Appraisal

There is strong empirical support for interventions based on the ABA model in improving adherence to pediatric medical regimens, particularly those for chronic diseases (Meichenbaum & Turk, 1987; Rapoff & Barnard, 1991; Rapoff, 2000; Varni & Wallander, 1984). Interventions generated from an ABA perspective have primarily involved contingency management procedures, such as token systems. There does not appear to be any studies which have explicitly examined medical adherence from a rule-governed behavioral perspective, though this would seem feasible. For example, older children and adolescents with chronic diseases could be taught to identify unrealistic or unhelpful "rules" about medications (e.g., "Medications can be taken depending on how one feels.") and challenge these rules by verbal and experiential means (as with traditional cognitive therapy methods).

Despite strong empirical support, ABA approaches have been criticized on the following grounds: (1) The ABA model is too simplistic to account for the richness and complexity of human behavior. It is based on studies which modify the "... rate of trivial responses emitted by animals in barren controlled settings" (Bandura, 1995, p. 185) or what has been referred to as the "behavior of small animals in boxes" (Todd & Morris, 1992, p. 1441). This criticism underlies many which follow here and partly reflects the foundational work on operant conditioning with simpler organisms in highly controlled experimental settings. Not surprisingly, behaviorists have countered that research with simpler organisms can reveal basic processes (as in medical research) but acknowledge that elaborations and extensions are needed when moving to the study of more complex organisms (Skinner, 1974; Todd & Morris, 1992). They would also point to an extensive and diverse body of applied literature that speaks to the utility of ABA approaches in addressing socially significant problems in medicine, education, business, family life, and community settings (see Kazdin, 2000 and representative issues of the *Journal of Applied Behavior Analysis*); (2) Concerns have also been raised that "external" or "extrinsic" rewards may undermine "intrinsic" motivation (Deci & Ryan, 1985). For example, highly adherent patients may become nonadherent when offered external rewards for adhering to medical treatments. A variant of this criticism is voiced by parents who sometimes object to providing external rewards for something their child "should do" without being explicitly rewarded. Behavior analysts have addressed this issue and concluded that detrimental effects of rewards are rare, easily avoided, and they agree that more "natural" reinforcers are preferable (Eisenberger & Cameron, 1996); (3) The "cognitivist challenge" to the ABA model contends that human beings respond to "cognitive representations" of the environment and not the environments per se (Mahoney, 1974). ABA theory is criticized for minimizing or rejecting the causal role of cognitions and other "private events" (such as feelings and sensations) in human functioning (Bandura, 1996). ABA adherents counter with an oft-quoted remark by Skinner (1974): "What is inside the skin, and how do we know about it? The answer is, I believe, the heart of radical behaviorism" (pp. 211–212). Though they recognize that behavior analysts have traditionally ignored the study of private events, they also cite recent theoretical and empirical developments that seek to rectify this situation, such as relational frame theory and acceptance and commitment therapy (Anderson, Hawkins, & Scotti, 1997; Hayes, Strosahl, & Wilson, 1999; Wilson, Hayes, & Gifford, 1997); and (4) ABA approaches have been characterized as manipulative, totalitarian, and punitive (Todd & Morris, 1992). Some have even argued that it denigrates freedom and undermines personal agency (Bandura, 1997). The counter to this criticism is that controlling influences are omnipresent and need to be delineated so people can understand and counter these influences (Skinner, 1974). Also, behavior analysts have argued for greater use of positive reinforcement-based procedures and have actively worked to reduce aversive control and safeguard the rights of vulnerable groups, such as children and individuals with disabilities (Kazdin, 1994; Todd & Morris, 1992).

Clinical Implications of ABA Theory

Consider the example of a 14-year-old male who was diagnosed with polyarticular JRA 2 years ago. His disease has been under poor control as evidenced by multiple active joints, extended joint stiffness in the morning, severe limitations in daily activities, and moderate to severe joint pain reported by the patient. His regimen consists of an oral anti-inflammatory medication (Naproxen) two times a day, range of motion exercises once per day, and wearing joint splints on his wrists at night. The referring rheumatologist suspected that nonadherence to this regimen contributed significantly to the patient's poor disease control. The patient lived with both parents, who worked outside the home, and an older sister.

Applying an ABA perspective to this case might suggest the following strategies:

- Focusing on the complexity of the regimen (response costs), the clinician might discuss with the patient's physician and occupational therapist ways to simplify the regimen. For example, the patient may be able to switch to another anti-inflammatory medication (Feldene) that is taken once per day rather than twice and reduce the number of range-of-motion exercises.
- The clinician's assessment might reveal that the patient tends to be more adherent to his regimen on days when he has increased joint pain and stiffness. On these days, his symptoms "remind him" to take his medications, do his exercises, and wear his splints. The clinician might need to help the patient and parents find specific and reliable cues or prompts for adherence on days when his disease symptoms are not as severe. For example, the patient may be asked to monitor and record adherence tasks as he completes them using a calendar chart posted in a prominent place or use a daily pill box.
- Considering potential negative regimen effects, the clinician may need to provide advice about how to reduce aversive consequences of adhering to the regimen. For example, anti-inflammatory drugs often cause gastric irritation and pain. The patient could be reminded to take medications with foods and along with his parents, to consult with his physician about the use of antacid medications to reduce gastric irritation and pain.

- Attending to potential positive consequences for adherence, sometimes these occur for this patient when he is symptomatic and adherence results in relief of disease symptoms, such as pain. During relatively asymptomatic periods, positive consequences may need to be specifically programmed to reinforce adherence behaviors. For example, the patient could be exposed to a token system program, whereby he earns points for adhering to regimens tasks and exchanges points for routine and special activities. The token system might also need to include point fines for nonadherence.
- Taking a rule-governed perspective, the patient may operate on unrealistic or unhelpful rules about his disease and regimen. For example, he may think he needs to be vigilant about following his regimen only when he is symptomatic. The clinician would need to help him challenge the utility of this rule and to formulate more helpful rules to advance his health status (e.g., "I need to take my medications, do my exercises, and wear my splints at night, even when I feel ok, in order to control my arthritis and to prevent flare-ups.").

Summary and Implications of Adherence Theories

At the theoretical and philosophical level, there may be little hope (or need) for agreement between proponents of different theories about why people do or do not follow prescribed medical regimens. Proponents of competing theories ". . . practice their trades in different worlds" and communication across the theoretical divide is "inevitably partial" (Kuhn, 1970, pp. 149–150).

Agreement can be reached about the content and behavior change processes addressed by various theories. The content refers to the focus on adherence behaviors or what people actually do in relation to a prescribed regimen (even within the TRA/BP, the intermediary step of "intentions" leads to adherence-related behavioral requirements). Behavior change processes can be summarized as two basic types: (1) cognitive or self-mediated thought processes (e.g., self-efficacy in Bandura's theory and rule-governed behavior in ABA) and (2) environmental contingencies (e.g., cues to action in the HBM and consequences in ABA). What clinicians do to activate these processes is similar despite differing theoretical frameworks and constructs. That is, clinicians can promote adherence to medical regimens by:

- Verbally persuading patients and their families of the value of prescribed regimens.
- Providing competent role models who demonstrate how to successfully manage regimens.
- Helping patients and families set specific goals and monitor progress to these goals.
- Teaching patients and families the necessary skills for carrying out regimen tasks.
- Helping patients and their families arrange more reinforcing consequences for adherence, be they direct, vicarious, or self-generated.

Those of different theoretical persuasions may have more in common than they thought. Clinicians and researchers should direct their energies and talents to applying generic principles and strategies, while retaining their unique perspectives and cherished theoretical constructs. Patients and their families would be better served by taking this integrative approach.

Chapter 4
Measurement Issues: Assessing Adherence and Disease and Health Outcomes

It is vital to assess adherence because adherence failure is a ubiquitous problem that directly impacts the health and well-being of children. This chapter will expand on reasons *why* to assess adherence, as well as, *what* is to be assessed, *who* should be assessed (and who should do the assessment), and *how* to assess. Because there is no ideal measure of adherence, the most common methodological limitations and problems (such as measurement reactivity) will be reviewed and strategies for minimizing their impact will be offered. Medical outcomes (such as glycosylated hemoglobin levels in patients with diabetes) are often treated as indirect measures of adherence, even though they are separate phenomena with a variable and conditional relationship to adherence. Measures of disease or health-status outcomes, including quality of life measures, will be reviewed separately.

Why Assess Adherence?

The aims or functions of adherence assessment are consistent with those applicable to assessing any behavioral phenomenon: (1) screening or diagnosis; (2) prediction; (3) selection of intervention strategies; and (4) evaluation of intervention efforts (Barrios, 1988; Johnston & Pennypacker, 1993; Mash & Terdal, 1988).

Screening and Diagnosis

Not all patients are candidates for interventions to improve medical adherence. Clinicians may do more harm than good if they intervene with those patients who are maintaining an acceptable level of adherence (Finney, Hook, Friman, Rapoff, & Christophersen, 1993). Patients may require varying degrees of assistance to elevate their adherence levels. Screening is helpful in determining who would benefit from efforts to modify adherence and to limit the time and expense of monitoring and intervening with patients who do not require assistance. This could be done by monitoring adherence in a group of patients, setting a minimum criterion for nonadherence (e.g., <80% of medications taken), and offering interventions to those classified as nonadherent.

M.A. Rapoff, *Adherence to Pediatric Medical Regimens*, Issues in Clinical Child Psychology, DOI 10.1007/978-1-4419-0570-3_4,
© Springer Science+Business Media, LLC 2010

In some cases, a specific "diagnosis" of nonadherence is required. The Diagnostic and Statistical Manual of Mental Disorders (DSM-IV) contains a supplementary (or "V") code labeled "Noncompliance with Treatment" (American Psychiatric Association, 1994). To make this diagnosis requires the clinician to identify adherence problems that are severe enough to require independent clinical intervention. This, in turn, requires some measure of adherence and specific criteria to determine the severity of adherence problems (neither of which are specified in the code description). If this code could be further defined and standardized, clinicians who provide adherence interventions could be reimbursed by third-party payers for their efforts. Also, patients and their families, who do not warrant other (possibly more stigmatizing) psychiatric diagnoses, could avoid unnecessary out-of-pocket expenses to receive assistance in improving adherence.

Prediction

Isolating predictors of adherence requires an adequate measure of adherence. Also, the best predictor of future adherence to a specific regimen is current or past adherence to that same regimen (confirming the old maxim that the best predictor of future behavior is past behavior). Adherence has also served as a predictor of disease and health-status outcomes. Thus, adequate assessments of adherence, along with disease-status information, measures of psychosocial adjustment, and properties of the prescribed regimen, can facilitate better predictions about the outcomes of various medical treatments.

Intervention Selection

Adherence assessment can aid in the selection of intervention strategies for improving adherence. In designing adherence interventions, clinicians need to know the extent and nature of adherence problems. Those patients with less severe adherence problems would require less complex efforts to improve adherence. For example, patients who occasionally forget to take medications may be provided with simple strategies to prompt adherence (such as setting a watch alarm). In contrast, those patients who frequently miss doses and actively resist their parents' attempts to prompt adherence might need a more complex intervention, involving prompting, shaping, reinforcement, and even mild punishment (e.g., time-out) strategies.

The nature of adherence problems may dictate the type of intervention needed. Patients who underdose (the most common medication-adherence error) may require a different intervention (e.g., instructing them about the importance of maintaining a therapeutic drug level to optimize treatment benefits) than those who overdose (e.g., instructing them to avoid trying to make up missed doses by taking extra doses). Expanding assessments to include a functional analysis of variables that impact adherence (such as antecedent and consequent events) would greatly enhance the ability of clinicians to select individualized interventions that match the unique history and life circumstances of their patients.

Evaluation of Intervention Efforts

Adequate assessments of adherence are necessary to evaluate efforts to improve adherence to medical treatments. The relative efficacy of different approaches to improving adherence can be evaluated, such as educational vs. behavioral strategies. Clinicians can also determine whether adherence interventions can be successfully faded out or modified if they fail to address adherence problems. Adherence assessments are also needed to evaluate the efficacy or effectiveness of medical treatments. If adequate adherence can be demonstrated, then the relative merits of various medical treatments can be more accurately determined in clinical and research contexts.

What Is to Be Assessed? Selection of Target Behaviors

Adherence is about behavior. But which behaviors are selected for assessment depends on the type of illnesses and their associated treatments. For acute illnesses (such as otitis media), "medication taking" is the primary behavior of interest, such as the ingestion of antibiotics on a specific schedule (from 1 to 4 times a day) over a limited period of time (5–14 consecutive days). The situation is more complex for chronic disease regimens. These regimens require multiple and more complex classes of behaviors over an extended or indefinite period of time. Therefore, they require more complex and long-term assessments of adherence.

Given these multicomponent regimens, which behaviors in a complex regimen should be selected for assessment? Guidelines for target behavior selection from the behavioral assessment literature offer some clues (Barrios, 1988; Friman, 2009; Kratochwill, 1985; Mash & Terdal, 1988; Sturmey, 1996).

Guidelines for Selecting Target Regimen Behaviors

(1) *Select them all (or at least baseline them all).* This means selecting all behaviors relevant to adhering to a particular treatment regimen. The rationale for this strategy is that there is currently no empirical basis for selecting one behavior over another in terms of its importance in achieving medical treatment goals. In theory, they are all considered equally important and need to be assessed.

Although in theory all regimen behaviors should be given equal weight, this does not seem to be the case in clinical practice. Providers seem to emphasize certain regimen components over others (e.g., medications), possibly because they consider these components more critical to treatment success or because they have more expertise in and responsibility for certain components (e.g., medication management for physicians). The choice of which regimen behaviors to select for measurement may depend on providers' judgments of which regimen behaviors are critical to the health of their patients.

A variant of this approach would be to conduct baseline or screening assessments of all relevant regimen behaviors and then target low-rate behaviors or ones that fail to meet some minimum standard (e.g., <80% adherence) for further assessment and intervention. This would establish some empirical basis for selecting target behaviors, but minimum standards of adherence (other than arbitrary ones) have not been determined for most pediatric medical regimens.

(2) *Select behaviors that are identified as most problematic or disturbing to others.* With reference to medical-adherence issues, these "others" are most often parents and providers. The patients themselves may not acknowledge problems with adherence. Interviewing parents or providers can reveal which behaviors need to be the focus of assessment. Most likely, these will be behaviors perceived as critical to the patient's health and those that have been difficult to establish or maintain for a particular patient. This guideline would appear to be the most socially or ecologically valid as it addresses the specific concerns of patients and other key people (family members and providers).

(3) *Select critical or "keystone" behaviors.* Originally, "keystone" behaviors were described as those behaviors that produce response generalization; i.e., altering the keystone behavior would produce desirable changes in other target behaviors (Sturmey, 1996). Some behaviors are chained together or may be part of the same functional class, such as insulin injections in relation to eating and exercise for patients with diabetes. Altering one behavioral requirement may produce changes in other behaviors. However, adherence to different behavioral requirements (such as diet, exercise, and medication taking) within the same treatment regimen may not be highly correlated (Johnson, 1993). Thus, altering one behavior may fail to produce changes in other relevant behaviors.

The general concept of keystone or critical behaviors, however, might prove useful. Providers who treat patients with chronic diseases prescribe a myriad of behaviors which (hopefully) to the best of their knowledge and experience are likely to improve the health and well-being of their patients. The key in selecting keystone behaviors is to identify which of these behaviors are critical to optimal medical-treatment outcomes. These critical regimen behaviors can be gleaned from medical textbooks, surveys of relevant providers, and consensus treatment guidelines from governmental and medical associations that set empirically validated criteria for standard medical practice (Johnson, 1993). For example, consistency in taking inhaled corticosteroids in the treatment of moderate to severe asthma may be more critical for reducing morbidity and mortality for large numbers of patients than environmental control measures, such as minimizing indoor allergens. Even if critical behaviors can be identified for groups of patients with a particular disease, they may not be relevant for a particular patient.

(4) *Select behaviors that are the easiest to change.* The rationale for this guide-line is that behaviors that are more easily changed can create momentum to change, other, more difficult behaviors. This approach would help patients be more successful in managing their illness and should enhance their self-efficacy.

Who Should Be Assessed and Who Should Assess?

Adherence assessment in pediatrics is arguably more complex than in adult medicine, in that others (particularly parents) have varying degrees of responsibil-ity in helping children carry out medical regimens. In fact, for younger children, parents are primarily or exclusively responsible for ensuring that treatments are consistently maintained. Therefore, the focus needs to be on assessing patient and parent regimen-related behaviors. For school-aged children, this might also involve assessing the behaviors of school nurses who supervise and/or sometimes administer treatments at school.

A variety of informants or assessors can be employed to monitor adherence. These include parents, physicians, nurses, and therapists. There are obvious advan-tages to employing these significant others. They are often a major source of data on adherence because of their unique and regular access to patients in their homes, schools, clinics, and in the community. In research contexts, data obtained from par-ticipant observers or raters need to meet rigorous criteria of validity, reliability, and accuracy, as with data from other sources (Johnston & Pennypacker, 1993). This requires proper training and quality controls. For example, in some of our clinical studies on improving adherence to medication regimens for pediatric rheumatic dis-eases, my colleagues and I trained parents to conduct observations or pill counts and the parents obtained acceptable levels of agreement with independent observers (Pieper et al., 1989; Rapoff, Lindsley, & Christophersen, 1984; Rapoff, Purviance, & Lindsley, 1988a, 1988b).

How to Assess Adherence? A Critical Review of Assessment Strategies

A variety of strategies exist for assessing adherence, including assays, observations, electronic monitors, pill counts, provider estimates, and patient/parental reports (Farmer, 1999; Quittner, Espelage, Ievers-Landis & Drotar, 2000). Each of these strategies has associated assets and liabilities, including relative costs and clinical applicability or feasibility (see Table 4.1). Some liabilities are common to all these measures and will be discussed later in this chapter. Also, some of these strategies are only applicable to certain types of regimens, such as assays to assess medication adherence.

Table 4.1 Assets and liabilities of adherence measures

Measure	Assets	Liabilities
Assays	Verify drug ingestion	Pharmacokinetic variations
	Adjust drug levels	Short-term measure
	Quantifiable	Invasive and expensive
Observation	Direct measure of nonmedication regimens	Obtrusive and reactive
		Clinically impractical
	Repeated measurements	Difficult to obtain representative samples
	Necessary to functional assessment	
Electronic monitors	Precision (reveals dosing and dosing-interval data)	Does not measure consumption
	Continuous and long-term assessments	Reactive
	Help identify drug reactions	Mechanical failures
Pill counts	Feasible	Relies on patients to return unused medications
	Inexpensive	
	Validate provider or patient estimates	Overestimates adherence
		Does not measure consumption
Provider estimates	Feasible	Overestimates adherence
	More accurate than global patient reports	Accuracy not a function of provider training or experience
	Correctly identifies adherent patients	Global estimate
Patient report	Feasible	Overestimates adherence
	Accurate if patient is asked in nonjudgmental fashion	Subject to reporting bias ("faking good")
	Patient has continuous access to own behavior	Not feasible for younger children

Drug Assays

Description. Laboratory assays can measure drug levels, metabolic products of drugs, or markers (pharmacologically inert substances or low-dose medications) added to target drugs in bodily fluids, such as serum, urine, and saliva (Roth, 1987). To properly interpret assays requires some basic knowledge of clinical pharmacokinetics, which is concerned with the absorption, distribution, and elimination of drugs in the body (for general and relatively nontechnical overviews, see Benet, Mitchell, & Sheiner, 1990; Johanson, 1992; Winter, 2003). The following is a simplified version of these processes and a description of other important terms relevant to interpreting drug assays.

Absorption of drugs depends initially on the dose administered and route of administration. Drugs can be delivered orally, parenterally (intravenous, intramuscular, or subcutaneous), by inhalation into the lungs, transdermally (skin patches), and via mucosal routes (the nose, mouth, or rectum). There are relative advantages and disadvantages of these various routes, such as immediate onset of action for intravenous vs. slow onset for oral routes (see Johanson, 1992, Table 2, p. 19 for a more thorough delineation). Because oral routes are most the common and relevant to assessing adherence, this discussion will focus on what happens when a drug has been administered orally.

Once a drug is administered, it enters the gastrointestinal tract where absorption takes place. At this point, absorption can be affected by the acidity in the stomach, contents of the stomach (such as food, which is why medications are often taken prior to meals), and the formulation of the drug (generic vs. brand versions). Metabolism of the drug primarily occurs in the liver as a result of enzymatic reactions. The rate or extent of metabolism can be affected by individual differences in the structure of liver enzymes (due to genetics) and the functioning of liver enzymes (which can be altered by a number of factors, including disease, age, and present or past administration of other drugs).

Once the drug has been absorbed and metabolized by the liver (so-called first-pass), it reaches the circulatory system where rapid distribution occurs to bodily tissues. Rapid distribution occurs because the blood circulates throughout the body every minute. Again, the liver comes into play, as there is a second pass through the liver after it is distributed throughout the body.

The next phase is elimination or excretion of the drug, which occurs primarily by the kidneys. Fluid is forced into the kidneys and contains the drug, its metabolites, other waste products (natural metabolites of bodily function) as well as electrolytes (such as potassium and sodium). That which is not needed or wanted by the body is transported out through the ureters to the bladder and eliminated through urination.

There are important concepts to consider when interpreting assays. The *bioavailability* of a drug is that percentage or fraction of the administered dose which enters the patients' systemic circulation (Winter, 2003). Several factors can affect bioavailability, including the intrinsic dissolution and absorption properties of a drug, the route of administration, the dosage form (tablet or capsule), the stability of the active ingredient of the drug in the gastrointestinal tract, and the extent of drug metabolism before reaching the circulatory system. The rate of elimination is directly related to plasma drug concentrations or the *half-life* of a drug, which is "...the amount of time required for the total amount of a drug in the body or the plasma drug concentration to decrease by one-half" (Winter, 2003). For most drugs in clinical situations, it can be assumed that the entire drug has been effectively eliminated after three to four half-lives (Winter, 2003).

Another important concept is *steady state* or when drug concentrations plateau, which is determined by the half-life of the drug. In general, it takes one half-life to reach 50% steady state, two half-lives to reach 75%, three half-lives to reach 87.5%, and four half-lives to reach 93.75%. It is also important to know maximum (*peak*) and minimum (*trough*) plasma levels for a given drug at steady state during a particular dosing interval. Plasma samples for drug assays are often drawn just before the next dose because trough levels are the most reproducible. Some drugs have a narrow therapeutic range and it is useful to identify fluctuations in plasma drug levels between doses. This is particularly true when the dosing interval is longer than the half-life, which results in large fluctuations in plasma drug levels (Winter, 2003).

Assets. Assays confer several advantages. They are quantifiable, clinically useful for determining subtherapeutic, therapeutic, and toxic levels of drugs, and they provide information on dose–response relationships (Rand & Wise, 1994). Also, they do not rely on potentially biased or inaccurate reports or estimates provided by patients, family members, or providers. Most importantly, assays confirm that drugs have been ingested. Chemical markers or tracers share these same advantages and can used with drugs for which there are no standard assays. Ideal markers should be chemically inert, nontoxic, nonradioactive, and undetectable by patients (Insull, 1984). Several types of chemical markers have been safely used for medication adherence assessments in pediatrics, such as riboflavin (Cluss & Epstein, 1984) and deuterium oxide (Rodewald, Maiman, Foye, Borch, & Forbes, 1989).

Liabilities. Assays have some serious limitations. They measure adherence over relatively short time intervals and thus fail to provide information about consistency in medication adherence over extended periods of time. Most assays reflect medication ingestion that has occurred (at best) no further back than five half-lives (Rudd, 1993). Take for example, the drug phenobarbital, which is a barbiturate used to treat seizure disorders. The plasma half-life of phenobarbital in children may be as short as 2–3 days (Winter, 2003). Assuming the half-life is 3 days (a more forgiving estimate than 2 days) and an assay reflects adherence no further back than five half-lives, a particular assay for phenobarbital would (at best) quantify adherence over the 15-day period prior to the assay assessment.

Assays can also be expensive and invasive, which makes them less feasible for use in pediatric settings (especially for chronically ill children who do not want another, and from their perspective, an unnecessary painful procedure like having their blood drawn). When assays are obtained in relation to dosing, it is also a complicating factor. Samples for assays are usually drawn just before the next medication dose (at trough levels), which requires knowledge of when the last dose was taken, which in turn depends on the accuracy of patient reports of when they took their most recent dose (Backes & Schentag, 1991). Laboratory errors can also be made in transporting, analyzing, and reporting results to providers, although these are considered to be minimal.

Low drug levels can also reflect inadequacies in the prescribed regimen. This may be particularly true for adolescents when medication doses are not adjusted for rapid growth (especially increased body fat for females and muscle mass for males) and hormonal changes that occur during puberty (Brooks-Gunn & Graber, 1994; Cary, Hein, & Dell, 1991).

Finally, pharmacokinetic variations in the way drugs are absorbed, metabolized, and excreted can account for variability in drug levels unrelated to or in addition to adherence. Such factors include the route of administration, the type of preparation (enteric coated, uncoated, or liquid forms), contents of the stomach, drug interactions, smoking, gastric pH levels, age, gender, puberty, body fat, and disease states, particularly compromised liver or renal functioning (Backes &

Schentag, 1991; Johanson, 1992; Winter, 2003). This is further complicated by the paucity of quantitative data in pediatrics (relative to adult medicine) on the relationship between pharmacokinetics and drug-treatment effects (Boréus, 1989).

Markers share some of the same disadvantages as standard assays, in terms of being affected by pharmacokinetic variations. Plus, adding markers to existing drugs may require approval by the FDA as a "new" drug and patients may consume foods that contain markers, such as riboflavin (Rudd, 1993).

Observation

Description. Direct observation of patient adherence is rare (Rapoff & Barnard, 1991). This may be because most studies examine adherence to medications and other measures, such as assays, are firmly entrenched as the optimal way to assess medication ingestion. Observation measures, in the form of behavioral checklists, have been used to evaluate patient technique in performing skills necessary for adherence. Behavioral checklists have been developed for assessing blood or urine glucose testing (Epstein, Figueroa, Farkas, & Beck, 1981; Wing et al., 1986), insulin administration (Gilbert et al., 1982), factor replacement therapy (Sergis-Davenport & Varni, 1983), and metered dose inhaler (MDI) use (Boccuti, Celano, Geller, & Phillips, 1996). Figure 4.1 provides an example of a behavioral checklist to monitor MDI technique for children with asthma. Of course, observing and evaluating how patients execute these skills says nothing about how often or consistently they accurately perform them.

Some studies have utilized parent or sibling observations as a primary data source, with acceptable levels of agreement with independent observers (Lowe & Lutzker, 1979; Rapoff et al., 1984). Direct and unobtrusive observations in camp settings have also been used to measure dietary adherence (Lorenz et al., 1985) and demonstrate concurrent validity of 24-h recall interviews (Reynolds, Johnson, & Silverstein, 1990).

Assets. Unlike other strategies, observational measures are direct measures of regimen-related behaviors. They are automatically valid, in the sense that they measure what they intend to measure (Johnston & Pennypacker, 1993). By directly measuring behavior, observational measures avoid subjective and potentially misleading judgments about behavior inherent in patient, family, and provider ratings of adherence. Observational measures also assess important dimensions of adherence behaviors, such as frequency (e.g., how often patients exercise), duration (e.g., the amount of time patients' exercise), interresponse time (e.g., the schedule or time between medication doses taken), and how well the behavior was performed (e.g., the way exercises were done or medications delivered relative to performance standards). Finally, by focusing on public behaviors, observational measures can also reveal contemporaneous controlling variables (antecedents and consequences) related to adherence that may be amenable to intervention (Mash &

Critical Skills
1. Spacer is correctly assembled (assembly criterion is specific to each spacer) (O,A,I)*
2. Patient opens InspirEase bag (I)
3. Canister is placed into actuator (O,A,I)
4. Patient closes mouth around mouthpiece (O,A,I)
5. Patient positions hand with index fingers on top of canister and thumb on bottom of
     spacer/mouthpiece (if child is physically unable to perform this skill, the parent can actuate
     the canister or another adaptation can be made) (O,A,I)
6. Patient presses canister once (O,A,I)
7. Patient actuates canister just before or at beginning of inhalation (O,A)
8. Patient continues to hold canister down through the entire inhalation (O)

Additional Skills
9.   Patient shakes canister at least 3 times (Prior to actuation) (O,A,I)
10. Patient exhales before inhalation (O,A)
11a. Patient inhales slowly and deeply through the mouth (O,A)
11b. Patient breathes in slowly (so that whistling does not sound), causing bag to deflate
      completely (I)
12. Patient holds breath to count of five (O,A,I)
13. Patient breathes back into bag, then breathes in slowly (so that whistling does not sound),
      causing bag to deflate completely (I)
14. Patient holds breath again to count of five (I)

Fig. 4.1 A metered-dose inhaler checklist.*Letters in parentheses indicate if items are appropriate
for different types of inhalers, with O = Optihaler, A = Azmacort, and I = InspirEase. Items are
not weighted equally. Failure to perform any of the critical skills (the number of these skills varies
by type of inhaler) results in a total score of zero. Reprinted with permission from Bocutti et al.
(1996).

Terdal, 1988). But if observational measures have so much to offer, why are
they so infrequently used in medical adherence research and less so, in clinical
practice?

Liabilities. The major problem with observational measures is accessibility.
Clinicians or researchers simply do not have sufficient access to patients in order
to measure their behavior in any consistent or representative way. At best, they have
limited samples of behavior that may not reflect how patients typically behave in
relation to prescribed regimens. Also, observational measures can be labor intensive, as they require extensive training, monitoring, and recalibration or retraining
of observers (Mash & Terdal, 1988).

   An oft-cited disadvantage of observational measures is their potential for reactivity (Friman, 2009; Wildman & Erickson, 1977). That is, when patients are being
observed, they may behave in ways that are not typical and usually in a socially
desired direction (e.g., they may be more adherent). Compared to other assessment
strategies, it is conceivable that directly watching someone has the potential of being
more reactive than taking a blood sample, electronically monitoring their adherence, or asking them about adherence behaviors. However, reactivity is a potential
problem with all measures of adherence.

   Another type of reactivity is relevant to those conducting observations. When
observers are being monitored, the quality of their observations may be higher than

when they are not being monitored (Wildman & Erickson, 1977). Observer reactivity may be particularly critical when using participant observers (such as parents) who have a direct interest in what is going on.

Another concern with observational measures for researchers is observer "drift" or variations in how paired-observers record behavior over time. Over time, paired-observers tend to develop a consensus about how behaviors are defined and recorded, which may substantially change or drift from the original coding definitions (Wildman & Erickson, 1977). Checking interobserver agreement between pairs of observers will not detect this problem because drift produces adequate agreement, but with a corresponding decline in accuracy over time (Foster, Bell-Dolan, & Burge, 1988). Fortunately, there are many ways to minimize drift, including rotating pairs of observers, videotaping observation sessions and scoring them in random sequences, and retraining (Foster et al., 1988; Kazdin, 1977). There are a host of other observer, instrument, and subject variables to consider when conducting behavioral observations (see Bellack & Hersen, 1988; Kazdin, 1977; Mash & Terdal, 1988).

Electronic Monitors

Description. Technological advances in microprocessors have led to the development of electronic measures of adherence. Electronic monitors are now available to record and store information on the date and time of tablet or liquid medication removal from standard vials, removal of pills from blister packages, removal of pills from an electronic pillbox, actuation of metered-dose inhalers, blood glucose test results, and patient diary notations on adherence or other clinical events, such as pain levels (Cramer, 1991; Riekert & Rand, 2002; Urquhart, 1994). These monitors can store information in real-time for up to several months and can be downloaded into data files for analysis. This is one of the most exciting developments in adherence measurement, with some even calling electronic monitors the "new gold standard" (Cramer, 1995). Electronic monitors have been used to measure adherence to oral or inhaled medications in pediatrics (Blowey et al., 1997; Coutts et al., 1992; Gerson et al., 2004; Kruse & Weber, 1990; Lau et al., 1998; Maikranz et al., 2007; McQuaid et al., 2003; Matsui et al., 1992; Modi et al., 2006, 2008; Olivieri, Matsui, Hermann, & Koren, 1991; Olivieri & Vichinsky, 1998; Rapoff et al., 2005; Walders et al., 2005). A task force review of evidence-based assessments in pediatric psychology concluded that electronic monitors were "well-established" measures of adherence (Quittner et al., 2008).

One such device for measuring removal of pills is the Medication Event Monitoring System (MEMS®) available from the AARDEX, Ltd., (Union City, CA). The hardware consists of two components: the monitor and communicator module. The monitor is a cap with self-enclosed electronic circuitry that fits on a standard pill vial. One version is the MEMS® TrackCap (with or without a child-resistant cap), which stores up to 3818 dose events and has a battery life of approximately 36 months. Another version is the MEMS® SmartCap (also available with or without a child-resistant cap), which stores up to 3818 dose events and has a battery life of about 18 months, but has two additional features: a visual display showing how many times the vial has been opened each day and how long (in hours) since the vial was last opened, as well as an optional audible signal programmed for when medications are to be taken. The communicator module is attached to a serial port of a computer and allows data from the cap to be downloaded into a software program that reads, displays, and prints out dosing records. Figure 3.2 shows a typical printout from an earlier version of the MEMS® for a child with JRA who participated in one of our studies on improving adherence to nonsteroidal anti-inflammatory medications (NSAIDS). The top portion of Fig. 4.2 shows the printout of her daily medication removal for a 1-week period and the bottom portion shows the calendar plot. This patient was prescribed Voltaren (a NSAID) on a twice daily schedule and the half-life of the drug was set at 14 h, in consultation with the treating rheumatologist. The printout shows the month (mm), day (dd), year (yy), hour (hh), minutes (mm), and seconds (ss) the cap was removed and the days, hours, and minutes that elapsed between openings. The calendar plot shows the number of times the cap was removed each day.

Several parameters can be obtained from the MEMS® (using data from Fig. 4.2): number and percent of doses removed (10 of 14; 71%); number and percent of optimal daily dosings (3 of 7 days where two doses were taken; 43%); an estimate of therapeutic coverage over the 7-day time course based on the half-life (76.3%); and the average and range of interdose intervals (based on 10 doses taken over 7 days, in this example, yields a mean interdose interval of 16.66 h and a range of 8.73–27.67 h, which can be compared to the ideal interval of 14 h). As can be seen, different results are obtained depending on the parameter used to reflect adherence. For example, using "percent of doses removed" (which is analogous to pill counts) yields a 71% adherence rate, in contrast to using "percent of optimal daily dosings," which yields a much lower adherence rate of 43%.

Assets. Electronic monitors provide a continuous and long-term measure of medication adherence in real-time, which is not available with any other measure. Monitors can reveal a spectrum of adherence problems, including (1) underdosing (the most common dosing error); (2) overdosing (which can contribute to toxic effects); (3) delayed dosing (dosing which exceeds recommended dosing intervals, which can reduce therapeutic coverage); (4) drug "holidays" (omitting doses for several days in succession without provider authorization); and (5) "white-coat" adherence or giving the appearance of adequate adherence by dumping medications or taking medications consistently several days before clinic visits (Riekert & Rand, 2002; Urquhart, 1994).

The close monitoring conferred by electronic devices can also help distinguish probable from improbable drug reactions or side effects. For example, a drug reaction reported by a patient (such as dizziness) can be correlated in real-time by an electronic monitor with inappropriate medication dosing, such as shortened intervals between doses or taking extra doses. Conversely, improbable drug reactions

Physician: Lindsley   Medication: Voltaren
Patient Name: Prescribed Regimen: BID
Medical Record Number: 004   Drug Duration Action: 14 hr.
Observation Period: Start: 10/10/92   00:01:00
                          Stop: 10/16/92   23:59:00
Total Recorded Events: 10   Events Listed for Time Zone: Central

Dose Time (Cap Removed)		Dose Interval (Elapsed Time)	Notes
mm/dd/yy	hh:mm:ss	dd:hh:mm	
10/10/92	07:22:40	0:13:58	
10/10/92	17:10:24	0:09:47	
10/11/92	20:50:40	1:03:40	E
10/12/92	05:34:56	0:08:44	
10/12/92	17:13:36	0:11:38	
10/13/92	05:57:20	0:12:43	
10/14/92	05:41:52	0:23:44	E
10/14/92	20:10:08	0:14:28	E
10/15/92	21:14:40	1:01:04	E
10/16/92	16:04:48	0:18:50	E

Notes Legend:
E - Dose Interval EXCEEDS Drug Duration of Action
F - Dose Time FILTERED due to less than 15 minutes separation from previous Dose Time
I - Dose Time INSERTED at end of Cap Open Length greater than 2 hours

October 1992

Date	Monday	Tuesday	Wednesday	Thursday	Friday	Saturday	Sunday
				--	--	--	--
5	--	--	--	--	--	2	1
12	2	1	2	1	1	--	--
19	--	--	--	--	--	--	--
26	--	--	--	--	--	--	--

Therapeutic   76.3%   Coverage:

Fig. 4.2 Example of data from an electronic monitor (MEMS)

can be revealed if the patient reports a side effect when the monitor indicates low adherence (Rudd, 1993).

Monitors can also help identify "actual" drug resistance (low efficacy in spite of high adherence to an adequate dosing regimen) vs. "pseudo" resistance due to delayed or underdosing (Rudd, 1993). Combined with plasma assays, monitors can also help identify within-patient variation in plasma concentrations, as they provide information about the timing of drug administration (Rubio, Cox, & Weintraub, 1992).

Finally, the detailed information on adherence patterns provided by electronic monitors can be used clinically to provide feedback and counseling to patients and their families during brief clinic visits or by telephone (Cramer, 1995).

Liabilities. When referring to the capability of electronic monitors, it is more precise to say that they measure "presumptive" dosing. The presupposition here is that patients ingest what they dispense. Thus, the major drawback of electronic monitors is that they generally do not confirm ingestion or proper inhalation of medications and may overestimate actual adherence. Assays are needed to help confirm ingestion (Roth, 1987). Although deliberate falsification can occur if patients dispense but fail to ingest medications, this seems highly unlikely as patients must do this at the precise time when medications are to be taken (Urquhart, 1994). Thus, the degree of effort needed to falsify adherence would seem to present adherence problems in its own right. Monitors could also underestimate adherence if patients take out several doses at once to carry with them when they are away from home or to load pill reminder boxes.

Electronic monitors, like any mechanical device, can malfunction. They may record events that did not occur, fail to record events that did occur, or simply stop working because batteries expired. However, most of these mechanical failures occurred with prototypes (Averbuch, Weintraub, & Pollock, 1990). Sometimes failures occur when devices are used in ways not designed by the manufacturers. For example, in a study monitoring prophylactic penicillin adherence among a sample of children with sickle cell disease, the investigators used liquid medications for some children and it penetrated into the device resulting in loss of data (Berkovitch et al., 1998). The clinical utility or feasibility of monitors is limited by the relatively high costs for the rental or purchasing of monitors, communicators, and proprietary software. There have also been unexpected mechanical failures of monitors (Berkovitch et al., 1998; Matsuyama, Mason, & Jue, 1993). Some of these failures may be patient induced, such as in our JRA adherence study when one 9-year-old female patient returned a completely demolished monitor with the explanation that an "entertainment center fell on it" (we suspected something more deliberate, such as a hammer wielded by the patient).

There are also practical problems regarding the convenience and portability of the monitors. The monitors are somewhat oversized and heavier relative to standard vial caps, which may make them cumbersome, particularly for patients on t.i.d. or q.i.d. dosing schedules that have to transport them outside the home. Also, in order to download data from the monitors, they have to be retrieved and in some cases, patients have lost the monitors or have not returned them. Ethical objections can also be made to using electronic monitoring ("big brother is watching"), particularly if patients are not informed about the capabilities of monitoring devices. This is particularly critical for children who are not afforded the same degree of legal or ethical protection as adults. A major obstacle in the past has been that patients are not willing to use electronic monitors for pills because they use a pillbox to help them be organized and remind them to take medications (Shellmer & Zelikovsky, 2007). There is now an electronic pillbox (MedSignals®, San Antonio, TX, USA) that has four bins for storing four different drugs, with each bin holding about 32 tables (the size of a 325 mg aspirin). The device also has multiple prompts for taking medications including an audible beep, flashing LED screen, and text messages on the screen. This device will be very helpful for researchers studying diseases, like HIV, that require multiple daily medications.

Pill Counts

Description. Pill counts have a long tradition in adherence assessment and are relatively straightforward. For example, consider the data from Fig. 4.2 on the patient prescribed Voltarin twice a day assessed over a 1-week period. Pill counts would involve counting medications at two points in times, separated by 1 week. The number of pills counted at time 2 (four pills on October 16, 1992) are subtracted from those counted at time 1 (14 pills on October 10, 1992) and this product (10 pills) is then divided by the total number of pills prescribed (14 pills) over the 1-week counting interval, to determine a fraction or proportion (0.71), which is then multiplied by 100 to obtain a percent of doses taken (thus, no. of pills removed ÷ no. of pills prescribed × 100, would be 10 ÷ 14 × 100 = 71%). Liquid medications can be similarly "counted" by measuring the volumes of medications at times 1 and 2. Another variation for inhaled medications is to weigh canisters at times 1 and 2 (Rand & Wise, 1994). Relative weights correlated with the number of actuations of the inhaler can be pretested with different types of canisters (e.g., to determine the initial weight of a full canister and progressive decreases in weight correlated with the frequency of actuations).

Assets. Pill counts are uncomplicated and relatively feasible for use in clinical settings. Their feasibility has been enhanced by obtaining pill counts from patients or family members by phone (e.g., Pieper et al., 1989). Because pill counts have been widely used in research, they can also be used to summarize and compare adherence rates to a wide variety of medication regimens and patient samples. Pill counts or measurements can also be used to validate other adherence assessment methods, such as patient, parent, or provider estimates.

Liabilities. Pill counts, like electronic monitors, cannot confirm ingestion. Most often, they overestimate adherence rates, which can occur if patients "dump" medications. Medications (particularly antibiotics) may also be shared with other family members. Pill counts also reveal very little about variations in drug administration, such as overdosing, underdosing, drug holidays, and the white-coat effect. Sometimes pill counts are not possible because patients do not bring medication containers to clinic visits, even when reminded by telephone calls prior to the visit. Patients may also dispense medications from more than one container or load them in pill-reminder containers ahead of time, thus precluding an accurate count (Rudd, 1993). Because of converging evidence that pill counts overestimate adherence relative to other methods (such as assays), some have recommended that investigators cease using this as a measure of adherence (Bond & Hussar, 1991).

Provider Estimates

Description. Provider estimates generally involve global ratings by physicians or nurses of the degree to which their patients are adherent to a particular regimen. For example, in one study, physicians were asked to rate adherence to medications, chest physiotherapy, and diet for children with cystic fibrosis using a 5-point Likert-type scale, with the endpoints being 4= "almost always (95% of the time)" and 0= "rarely (5% or less of the time)" (Gudas et al., 1991). Providers are sometimes asked to make dichotomous judgments (yes or no) about whether patients will be adherent.

Assets. Provider estimates are fast, simple, and inexpensive, which makes them very feasible for use in clinical practice. If providers assess adherence at all, they probably prefer this method. There is some evidence that provider estimates are better than global estimates obtained from patients or family members (Rapoff & Christophersen, 1982).

Liabilities. Provider estimates are not very accurate compared to other measures, such as assays (Rudd, 1993). Furthermore, providers are inaccurate in a specific way. Although they are generally accurate in identifying adherent patients, they often fail to identify nonadherent patients. This is nicely illustrated in one study where pediatric providers (nurses, resident, and staff pediatricians) were asked to predict which of their patients would be adherent to an antibiotic regimen for otitis media (Finney et al., 1993). In response to the question "Do you think this family will administer most of the prescribed medication?", providers' estimates were dichotomized as "will adhere" or "will not adhere." The "objective" measure of adherence was a pill count/liquid measurement conducted by the investigators in the patients' homes on the 7th to the 10th day of the prescribed regimen and the criterion for classifying patients as nonadherent was <80% of medicine removed. In this study, providers' predictions were treated as a diagnostic or screening test (like a laboratory test) and nonadherence, the condition to be diagnosed (like a disease). Viewing the findings this way yielded the following results: the *sensitivity* of provider predictions (the proportion of patients nonadherent by assay who were predicted to be nonadherent) was quite low (28%); the *specificity* of provider predictions (the proportion of patients adherent by assay who were predicted to be adherent) was perfect (100%); and the overall *accuracy* of provider predictions (proportion of all predictions, both positive and negative, that were correct) was moderate (65%). These results confirmed previous studies that show providers fail to identify patients who are nonadherent and illustrates that overall accuracy does not capture the type of prediction errors made by providers. Most importantly, it shows that a fair number of patients who could benefit from interventions to improve adherence would not be identified by their providers.

The inaccuracy of predictions or clinical judgment should come as no surprise to behavioral scientists and clinicians. There is good evidence that even among such "experts" in human behavior, clinical judgments are often biased and may be inferior to actuarial or statistical methods (Dawes, Faust, & Meehl, 1989).

Clinical judgments can be biased in a number of ways (Groopman, 2007; Rock, Bransford, Maisto, & Morey, 1987). Clinicians may hold on to or become "anchored" to their initial judgments even when faced with new and disconfirmatory evidence (the "anchoring" bias). Clinicians may also base judgments on the apparent correlation of two events (e.g., adherence and patient characteristics, like intelligence) when there is no direct correlation, the correlation is less than expected, or is the opposite of what is expected (the "illusory correlation" bias). Clinicians may also believe that judgment accuracy increases as they gain more clinical experience (the "overconfidence" bias). Finally, there is the "correspondence" bias, which is the generalized tendency for people to attribute other's behavior (but not their own behavior) to unique dispositional determinants (e.g., "laziness," "stupidity," or "lack of motivation"), while ignoring important situational determinants (see Gilbert & Malone, 1995 for an excellent review). All of these biases have the potential of reducing the accuracy of clinical judgments and experienced clinicians may actually be more vulnerable to their effects (Groopman, 2007; Rock et al., 1987).

An additional question is on what basis do providers make predictions or judgments about adherence? I queried several experienced pediatricians in private practice and pediatric residents and staff at our medical center and asked them if they make judgments about patient adherence and on what basis they made these judgments. They all agreed that they made such judgments (not surprisingly, given the focus of my inquiry). They based their judgments on several factors: (1) health or disease status (such as the presence of wheezing in a child with asthma or resolution of otitis media after treatment, although one pediatrician said "Some will get better, no matter what you do."); (2) patient or family characteristics (intelligence or "brightness," socioeconomic status, "willfulness" of the child, and age, particularly adolescence); (3) the parents' or patients' level of "interest" as determined by their attention to the doctor's advice and if they had a list of questions or sought out information on their child's symptoms; (4) direct questioning of patients and/or parents about adherence; (5) checking to see if prescriptions have been refilled and how often; and (6) an in-office demonstration of treatment efficacy to rule-out this as a cause of treatment failure and, by default, to rule-in the likelihood of nonadherence (e.g., pre- and postassessments of pulmonary function to evaluate the efficacy of inhaled bronchodilators for children with asthma).

The hall of fame catcher, Yogi Berra, once said "A guy ought to be very careful in making predictions, especially about the future." As clinicians and researchers, we should acknowledge the monumental task of trying to predict adherence behaviors and try to critically analyze the basis for our predictions.

Patient/Parental Reports

Description. Consistent with the emphasis on history taking in clinical practice, it is not surprising that patient and/or family reports are often used to assess adherence. Reporting formats include *global ratings, structured interviews and questionnaires,* and *daily diaries.*

Global ratings, like provider estimates, require that patients or parents rate adherence over unspecified or varying (and sometimes lengthy) time intervals. For example, parents might be asked, "In the last 2 months, was there any time he missed taking his pills for more than 1 day?" (Gordis et al., 1969). Parents might also be asked to rate their children's adherence on a weekly basis using a Likert-type scale, with 1 being "very nonadherent" to 5 being "very adherent" (Rapoff et al., 1988b).

Over the past decade, significant progress has been made in the development of *structured interviews and questionnaires* for assessing adherence. As can be seen in Table 4.2, these self-report measures have been developed to assess adherence to regimens for asthma, cystic fibrosis, diabetes, HIV, spina bifida, and transplantation. Most of these measures have parent and patient versions to obtain independent ratings from multiple respondents.

Daily diaries require patients or parents to record specific adherence behaviors over varying lengths of time using standard forms or are obtained by phone interviews. Portable hand-held computers allow patients to record adherence events or other clinical parameters, such as pain levels (Dahlström & Eckernäs, 1991; Palermo, Valenzuela, & Stork, 2004). An excellent example of a daily dairy method is the extension and validation of the 24-h recall interview (a standard dietary assessment technique), which has been refined and extended to assess adherence to diabetes regimens by Suzanne Bennett Johnson and her colleagues (see Johnson, 1995 for a review). This method involves assessing and quantifying adherence to 13 standard components of regimens for diabetes. Interviews are conducted separately with patients and parents over the phone. They report the day's events in temporal sequence, from the time the child awakens in the morning until retiring to bed, but the interviewer records only diabetes-related activities. To ensure representativeness, three separate interviews are conducted over a 2-week interval; on 2 weekdays and 1 weekend day. Interviews are restricted to the previous 24 h to minimize recall errors. Each interview takes about 20 min to complete (Freund, Johnson, Silverstein, & Thomas, 1991).

Each of the 13 adherence measures are constructed to yield a range of scores, with higher scores indicating relative nonadherence and scores close to zero indicating relative adherence. For example, *glucose testing frequency* is calculated based on an ideal frequency of four times per day, for a total possible frequency of 12 over the three interview days. The number of glucose tests reported is divided by the ideal and multiplied by 100 (e.g., $4 \div 12 \times 100 = 33$). This product is then subtracted from 100 (e.g., $100 - 33 = 67$), so that high scores indicate few glucose tests and low scores indicate frequent tests (e.g., a score of 67 indicates the patient reported four glucose tests being conducted over 3 days). This measure has also been adapted for

How to Assess Adherence? A Critical Review of Assessment Strategies

87

Table 4.2 Summary of reliability and validity information for structured interviews and self-report measures of adherence

Measure/authors	EBA classification	Number of items/respondent	Internal consistency	Test-retest reliability	Interrater reliability	Validity
			Asthma			
Family Asthma Management System Scale (FAMSS) (Klinnert et al., 1997; McQuaid et al., 2005)	Approaching well established	Semistructured interview; parents of children with asthma and with children (11–17 yrs old)	Total $\alpha = 0.84$	Not assessed	Intraclass correlations ranged from 0.67 to 0.93	Adherence scores significantly related to functional impairment/morbidity ($r = -0.39$), parent knowledge ($r = 0.36$), and child self-efficacy ($r = 0.36$). Adequate convergence with MDILog data ($r = 0.29$)
Disease Management Interview – Asthma (Modi & Quittner, 2006a)	Promising	28 items/parents and children >10 yrs.	Not assessed	Not assessed	Parent–child agreement: $r = 0.63$	Child self-report of adherence associated with no. of barriers to adherence ($r = -0.46$)

Table 4.2 (continued)

Measure/authors	EBA classification	Number of items/respondent	Internal consistency	Test-retest reliability	Interrater reliability	Validity
Cystic fibrosis						
Disease Management Interview-CF (DMI-CF) (formerly; treatment adherence questionnaire) (Quittner, Espelage et al., 2000)	Well established	51 items/parents and children over 10 years	Not assessed	$rs = 0.62$ to 0.73 (adolescent reports) $rs = 0.76$ to 0.88 (parent reports)	Parent–Teen Agreement: $r = 0.55$ nebulized meds $r = 0.78$ CPT Parent–child agreement: $r = 0.69$ nebulized meds $r = 0.88$ CPT	Not assessed
Treatment Adherence Rating Scale (TARS); (DeLambo, Ievers-Landis, Drotar, & Quittner, 2004)	Promising	16 items/parents and chil-dren/adolescents	Airway clearance/aerosolized medications $\alpha = 0.82$–0.84	$rs = 0.42$ to 0.57 among informants (adolescent, mother, father)	Not assessed	Not assessed
Diabetes						
Self-Care Adherence Interview (SCAI) (Hanson et al., 1989, 1996, 1992)	Approaching well established	15 items/semi structured interview/parents and adolescents (10–20 yrs)	Not assessed	3-month $r = 0.70$ 6-month $r = 0.68$–0.70 1-year $r = 0.71$	$r = 0.95$–0.98	Correlations between the SCI and glycemic control ranged from -0.20 to -0.28 in different samples

Table 4.2 (continued)

Measure/authors	EBA classification	Number of items/respondent	Internal consistency	Test-retest reliability	Interrater reliability	Validity
Self Care Inventory(SCI) (Davis et al., 2001; Delamater et al., 1997; Greco et al., 1990; La Greca, Swales, Klemp, & Madigan, 1988; Wysocki et al., 2000)	Well established	14 items/parents and adolescents	$\alpha = 0.76$ adolescent; $\alpha = 0.87$ parent	2-week $r = 0.77$	Not assessed	Good correlations reported between 24-h recall and SCI. Higher levels of self care (SCI) reportedly associated with better metabolic control
Diabetes Regimen Adherence Questionnaire (DRAQ) (Bond et al., 1992; Brownlee-Duffeck et al., 1987; Thomas, Peterson, & Goldstein, 1997)	Well established	15 items/adolescents (8–17 yrs)	Total $\alpha = 0.78$–0.80	Not assessed	Not assessed	Good correlations with health beliefs ($rs = 0.29$–0.33) and some social problem-solving skills ($rs = 0.43$–0.64)

Table 4.2 (continued)

Measure/authors	EBA classification	Number of items/respondent	Internal consistency	Test-retest reliability	Interrater reliability	Validity
			HIV/AIDS			
Pediatric AIDS Clinical Trials Group (PACTG): Adherence modules (Farley, Hines, Musk, Ferrus, & Tepper, 2003; Van Dyke et al., 2002)	Promising	2 Interview-administered Modules/parents and children (0–17 yrs old)	Not assessed	Not assessed	Not assessed	Mixed evidence regarding the association between the PACTG and virological response (90% sensitivity, 43% specificity, 69% positive predictive value)
			Spina bifida			
Parent Report of Medical Adherence in Spina Bifida Scale (PROMASB) (Holmbeck et al., 1998)	Approaching well established	39 items/parents of children with spina bifida	$\alpha > 0.65$ for 13 of 15 scales	Not assessed	Mother–father agreement: $r = 0.39$ total adherence scale Interrater reliability = 85%	Not assessed
			Transplantation			
Behavioral Affective and Somatic Experiences (BASES): Compliance Scale (Parent version) (Phipps, Hinds, Channell, & Bell 1994)	Approaching well established	38 items/compliance scale 8-items/parents of children who have undergone transplantation	Total $\alpha = 0.77$	Not assessed	Nurse–parent agreement: $r = 0.56$ median correlation	Not assessed

Table 4.2 (continued)

Measure/authors	EBA classification	Number of items/respondent	Internal consistency	Test-retest reliability	Interrater reliability	Validity
Self-Regulation of Medication Adherence Battery (SRMAAB) (Tucker et al., 2001)	Promising	10 items/patients who have undergone renal transplants (6–20 years old)	Not assessed	Not assessed	Not assessed	Sensitive to cultural differences in adherence between African-American and Caucasian patients.

EBA = Evidence Based Assessment

Note: Reprinted from Table 1, Quittner et al. (2008). Copyright 2008 by Society of Pediatric Psychology. Reprinted by permission of Oxford University Press.

assessing adherence to regimens for HIV (Marhefka et al., 2006; Naar-King, Fey, Harris, & Arfken, 2005). Strong stability coefficients, good parent–child agreement, and associations between adherence and glycemic control in diabetes and viral load in HIV have been reported for the 24-h recall interview (Quittner et al., 2008).

Another cued-recall daily diary method is the Daily Phone Diary (DPD), which was originally developed to assess daily activities of mothers and children with cystic fibrosis (Quittner & Opipari, 1994). Similar to the 24-h recall interview, parents and children are asked to reconstruct their previous day and each activity is recorded by an interviewer on a computer screen with clock hands that rotate through a 24-h clock, a set of activities, companions, and a rating scale for mood. Interviews are conducted on multiple (2 or 3) days with the primary caretaker and adolescent. The DPD has been adapted to assess adherence to regimens for asthma, cystic fibrosis, and HIV (Modi & Quittner, 2006b; Wiener, Riekert, Ryder, & Wood, 2004). The DPD has yielded high levels of interrater reliability and strong to modest convergence with self-report and electronic monitoring of adherence and has been negatively correlated with viral load in HIV (Quittner et al., 2008).

Assets. In general, patient or proxy (such as parents) reports are relatively simple, convenient, inexpensive, and clinically feasible (Bond & Hussar, 1991). They also address the problem of accessibility to patient behaviors over time and in ecologically relevant contexts (such as home and community).

How patients or family members are questioned about adherence may be critical in the quality of data obtained by reports. Questions that are nonjudgmental, specific, and time limited are likely to yield more accurate information about adherence, as they are less likely to generate evasive and defensive reactions and are less subject to recall errors or misunderstanding (Kaplan & Simon, 1990; Klinnert McQuaid, & Gavin, 1997; Rand, 2000). For example, contrast the following formats for questioning a parent about their child's adherence during a return clinic visit after a 10-day antibiotic course for otitis media:

> *Type A.* [**not recommended**]: "Mrs. Johnson, Nathan doesn't seem to be any better. Did you give him ALL of that medicine I prescribed?" (Said with a disapproving facial expression).
> Type B. [**recommended**]: "Mrs. Johnson, Nathan doesn't seem to be feeling any better. This can happen for many reasons. Sometimes a different or stronger medicine is needed. Sometimes a child doesn't get enough of the medicine. Many parents have problems giving medicines to their children; my husband and I sometimes forget to give our son his medicine when he's sick. I wonder if you have had any problems giving Nathan his medicine for one reason or another?" (Said in an empathetic, but not patronizing manner).

Although these two formats are admittedly characterizations, "Type A" is an invitation for parental defensiveness and incomplete or inaccurate disclosures about adherence, while "Type B" is more likely to elicit complete and accurate reports and lead to a dialogue about obstacles to adherence.

Diary and structured interviews offer additional advantages of providing detailed information on adherence patterns, the types of problems or obstacles encountered, and can be correlated with disease symptoms or outcomes. They can also be integrated into disease-management programs, which facilitate patient and family involvement in health care (Rand & Wise, 1994). Computerized diary or interview methods can also facilitate the disclosing of more sensitive information, such as adherence to safe-sex practices.

Dairy and structured interviews may be the best of the patient or family report measures because they are less labor-intensive for patients and families and more comprehensive. Evidence-based assessments of adherence measures have been reported using the criteria of "promising" (the measure is presented in at least one peer-reviewed article, is sufficiently described and available from the authors, and some vague or moderate statistics are presented on reliability and validity), "approaching well-established" (the measure is presented in at least two peer-reviewed articles, is sufficiently described and available from the authors, and some vague or moderate statistics are presented on reliability and validity), and "well-established" (the measure is presented in at least two peer-reviewed articles by different investigators, is sufficiently described and available from the authors, and statistics are presented indicating good validity and reliability in at least one peer-reviewed article) (Cohen et al., 2008a). The psychometric properties of the 24-h recall interview and DPD are strong and have led to the conclusion that they are "well-established" instruments for assessing adherence (Quittner et al., 2008). However, more work needs to be done to establish the psychometric properties of structured interviews, as they range from "promising" to "well-established" instruments for assessing adherence (Quittner et al., 2008).

Liabilities. Patient or family reports tend to overestimate adherence, most notably, by minimizing doses that have been missed. This is likely to be truer for global estimates vs. diaries or structured interviews. Global estimates can tax the person's memory for adherence events and lead to errors in self-reports (Tourangeau, 2000). Unless they are actively rehearsed, memories fade within a short period of time. The "outer limits" of recall for events are generally less than 2 weeks (Rudd, 1993). Also, people tend to remember unique events (ones that are stimulating or emotionally laden) and remember events in chronological order for up to 10 days and thereafter, in relation to other major events, such as holidays and birthdays. Diary methods can obviate the need for remembering events if patients complete them close in time to the behavior being monitored. However, about 50% of patients keep complete records (Johnson, 1993). Even if diaries are complete, one cannot ascertain when and where they were completed.

Report measures are also sensitive to demand or social desirability effects. That is, patients or families may tell providers what they want to hear, which could lead to overestimates or outright deception about adherence (Johnson, 1993). In this way, the patient or family "protects" their relationship with the provider or at least avoids their disapproval.

Proxy informants (such as parents) do not always have access to relevant behaviors, especially during adolescence. For example, only about 50% of diabetes-related activities are observed by parents (Johnson, 1995). Obviously, parents can only report on that which they see.

Daily dairy and structured interview methods appear to be the most promising of all the patient and family report measures. Parents and patients are interviewed separately to obtain more representative samples of adherence behaviors, and psychometric data on reliability and validity seem to meet minimal standards. However, further work is needed to corroborate these methods by more direct measures such as observations, assays, or electronic monitoring.

Comparative Performance of Adherence Measures

Compared to the adult literature, there are relatively few studies that have directly compared adherence measures with pediatric patients. The "classic" comparative assessment study in the pediatric literature was reported almost 40 years ago by Gordis et al. (1969). They compared patients' and their mothers' reports of adherence to penicillin prophylaxis for rheumatic fever with urine assays obtained during clinic visits, at least every 2 months for a 6-month period. Children were classified as compliers if they or their mothers' reported at $\geq 75\%$ of the visits that medication had been taken the day they were reporting. By urine assay, children were classified as *compliers* if $\geq 75\%$ or more of urine specimens were positive for penicillin, as *noncompliers* if $\leq 25\%$ of specimens were positive, and as *intermediate* compliers if 26–74% of specimens were positive. Using these criteria, 69–73% of patients were classified as compliers by patient/parental report, in contrast to 33–42% by urine assays. The major conclusion of this study was that patient or parental reports of adherence are "grossly inaccurate." Smyth and Judd (1993) compared parent reports with urine assays to assess adherence to antibiotic prophylaxis for pediatric patients with urinary tract infections. Although 97% of parents reported their children took antibiotics every day, only 69% of urine assays were positive. Another study on adherence to antibiotics for otitis media found significant correlations between parent interviews, parent diaries, volume measurements, and urine assays. However, correlations between urine assays and the other adherence measures were not significant for an antihistamine-decongestant medication (Devries & Hoekelman, 1988).

There are a group of studies that compare adherence rates obtained by electronic monitors to other measures of adherence (see Table 4.3). A consistent finding is that adherence rates are lower as measured by electronic monitors vs. rates obtained by pill counts, canister weighing, and parent or patient report. Also, bench studies of electronic monitors for metered dose inhalers, where investigators actuate devices and keep a record of actuations, have found high levels of accuracy (Apter, Tor, & Feldman, 2001; Julius, Sherman, & Hendeles, 2002).

Collectively, these studies and previous reviews of the literature suggest that assays or electronic monitors are superior measures of medication adherence

Table 4.3 Studies comparing electronic monitors (EM) to each other or to other measures of adherence in pediatric medicine

References	Sample/regimen	Comparison	Participants informed about EM capabilities?	Results	Comments
Apter et al. (2001)	MDI	Bench study, comparing three MDILog devices to diary record kept by investigators	N/A	Accuracy of MDILog for actuation of MDI = 97–100%; inhalation = 82–100%; shaking = 86–95%; late inhalations and multiple actuations = 97–99%	No artifactual recordings made by MDILogs during 3 days when carried in a bookbag; MDILog judged to be more accurate and reliable than previous versions
Bender, Milgrom, Rand, and Ackerson (1998)	N = 24 children (6–12 yrs) with asthma/inhaled beta-agonists and steroids	Metered-dose inhaler chronology (MDIC) compared to patient diaries	No	Complete use of corticosteroids (all doses taken) recorded on a median of 4.9% of days by MDIC vs. 54% by patient report; complete use of beta-agonists 12.7% by MDIC vs. 30% by patient report	Self-report distortion was correlated with lower parent education and affective responsiveness in family
Bender et al. (2000)	N = 27 children (7–12 yrs) with asthma/inhaled steroid	Parent and child self-report vs. canister weighing vs. Doser CT	Not reported	Mean adherence for parent and child report = >80%, for canister weighing = 69%, for Doser CT = 50%	Of the 301 Doser CT devices used in the study, 21% failed such that no data could be retrieved

Table 4.3 (continued)

References	Sample/regimen	Comparison	Participants informed about EM capabilities?	Results	Comments
Blowey et al. (1997)	$N = 19$ adolescents (12.5–17.9 yrs), post-renal trans-plant/cyclosporine	MEMS-4 compared to drug assays ($n = 14$) and physician or nurse and patient estimates	Yes	2 of 4 patients identified as nonadherent by MEMS had low cyclosporine levels (<50 ng/ml) and none of adherent patients; physician or nurse and patient estimates correctly identified 2 of 4 nonadherent patients	Mean adherence rate by MEMS = 91% (range 64–100%)
Butz, Donithan, Bollinger, Rand, and Thompson (2005)	$N = 157$ children with asthma (7–12 yrs)/inhaled steroid	Nebulizer monitor (Hill Rom, Inc.) vs. asthma diary cards	Yes	Concordance between diary and nebulizer monitor data was 85% agreement for use and nonuse	12 nebulizer monitor failures (8%); over four periods of time, return rates for diary data decreased from 75 to 44% compared to 92% usable Nebulizer monitor data

Table 4.3 (continued)

References	Sample/regimen	Comparison	Participants informed about EM capabilities?	Results	Comments
Chemlik and Doughty (1994)	$N = 20$ children and adults (11–72 yrs) with asthma/inhaled steroids and monitoring of peak flow rates	Nebulizer Chronolog (for inhaled steroids) and VMX Wright Mini-Log (for peak flow) vs. patient diaries	No	With diary recording errors defined as "…deviation of 10% or more in either direction from the actual reading or the recording of a phantom reading,": 52.5% error rate with diaries vs. Nebulizer Chronolog 17.5% error rate with diaries vs. Wright Mini-Log	73% of diary recording errors on inhaler use were overreporting of medication intake

Table 4.3 (continued)

References	Sample/regimen	Comparison	Participants informed about EM capabilities?	Results	Comments
Farley et al. (2003)	$N = 26$ (21 mos to 12.5 yrs) with HIV/antiretroviral medications	MEMS compared to pharmacy refill rates, caregiver self-report, physician/nurse assessment, and appointment keeping	Not reported	Sensitivity and specificity for predicting viral load were best for MEMS vs. other measures; combining MEMS and pharmacy refill rates resulted in highest sensitivity and specificity for predicting viral load; MEMS significantly correlated with pharmacy refill rates and physician/nurse assessments, but not caregiver report or appointment keeping	Adherence cutoff score of 80% derived from MEMS data predicted viral load (14 of 15 children with MEMS adherence rate >80% had an acceptable viral load) Adherence rates by MEMS ranged from 12.7 to 97.9% (Mdn = 81.4%)
Gibson, Ferguson, Aitchison, and Paton (1995)	$N = 29$ children (15 mos to 5 yrs) with asthma/prophylactic medications by MDI	Neubulizer Chronolog (NC300) compared to parent diaries	Yes	Mean daily adherence ($n = 22$) was 48% by NC300 vs. 72% by parent report	Significant drop (7%) in adherence during the last 20 days of study vs. first 20 days

Table 4.3 (continued)

References	Sample/regimen	Comparison	Participants informed about EM capabilities?	Results	Comments
Julius et al. (2002)	1, 2, and 4 puffs of fluticasone propionate MDI	Bench study of accuracy: 3 different electronic monitors (Doser CT, MDILog, and SmartMist) investigators actuated twice daily for 30 days with 2 units of each device and compared to date and time of actuation recorded in a log by investigators	N/A	Accuracy mean ($\pm$ SD): 100% for SmartMist; 94.3% $\pm$ 2.9% for Doser CT; 90.1% $\pm$ 6.9% for MDILog; there were no significant differences in accuracy between dosing schedules for any device	Additional actuations recorded by Doser CT and MDILog, with trend for decreasing accuracy over time (possibly due to battery decay?); Doser CT does not record date or time of each actuation and data cannot be downloaded to a computer; MDILog errors were "multiple dosing errors" (when an actuation is within 6–8 s of previous actuation)

Table 4.3 (continued)

References	Sample/regimen	Comparison	Participants informed about EM capabilities?	Results	Comments
Modi et al. (2006)	$N = 37$ children with cystic fibrosis (6–13 yrs)	MEMS vs. self-report, pharmacy refill history, and daily phone diaries	Not reported	A significant difference was found between parent-reported adherence and more objective measures, with parents reporting higher adherence rates compared to pharmacy refill, diaries, and electronic monitoring (p's < 0.05)	Parent report of adherence was 80% compared to 30–40% for pharmacy refill, diaries, and electronic monitoring
Modi and Quittner (2006b)	$N = 31$ children with cystic fibrosis; 30 children with asthma; subsample analyses conducted for measurement comparisons	Halolite™ vs. Daily Phone Diary (DPD); MDILogs vs. Daily Phone Diary	Not reported	Paired correlations between the DPD and Halolite™ for nebulized medications were 0.94 for frequency ($p = 0.001$) and 0.88 for direction ($p = 0.01$); the paired correlation for corticosteroids was 0.43 ($p = 0.22$) for DPD and MDILogs	

Table 4.3 (continued)

References	Sample/regimen	Comparison	Participants informed about EM capabilities?	Results	Comments
Milgrom et al. (1996)	$N = 24$ children (8–12 yrs) with asthma/inhaled beta-agonists and steroids	MDI Chronolog vs. patient diaries	No	Diary entries indicated median % of prescribed doses taken at 78.2% for beta-agonists and 95.4% for steroids vs. 48% and 32%, respectively, as recorded by MDI Chronolog	
Olivieri et al. (1991)	$N = 7$ patients (10–22 yrs) with transfusion-dependent homozygous β thalassaemia/oral chelating drug	MEMS vs. pill counts and patient diaries	No	Mean adherence by MEMS was 88.7% vs. 95.7% by pill counts and diaries	Delays (>60 min) in taking medication occurred on 55.6% of total days recorded by MEMS
Starr et al. (1999)	$N = 21$ adolescents with positive TB tests/isoniazid oral medication	MEMS vs. pill counts, urine assay, clinic attendance, and self-report	No	Mean adherence by MEMS was 66% vs. 91% by pill counts, 79% by assay, and 83% by clinic attendance; 65% of self-reports were inconsistent with MEMS data, generally overestimating adherence	Some patients did not bring MEMS device to clinic, resulting in incomplete data; metabolites of isoniazid are only present in the urine for 24 h after ingestion

compared to patient, parental, or provider reports and pill counts (Bond & Hussar, 1991; Quittner et al., 2008; Rand & Wise, 1994; Rapoff & Barnard, 1991; Rudd, 1993). However, there is no error-free way to assess adherence. All adherence measures share some common methodological problems that clinicians and researchers need to address.

Generic Methodological Issues and Recommendations for Adherence Measurement

Reactivity

All adherence measures are potentially subject to reactivity effects. If patients are informed about why someone is drawing their blood, watching them, asking them to use a special container with microelectronics, counting their pills, or asking them direct questions about adherence, they are more likely to behave in a socially sanctioned manner. Although reactivity can contribute to measurement error, it turns out to be useful in helping patients change their behavior, as with self-monitoring strategies to increase adherence. Fortunately, the behavioral observation literature would suggest that reactivity effects are either nonexistent or short lived and can be minimized (Johnston & Pennypacker, 1993; Wildman & Erickson, 1977). Clinicians and researchers can try to

- Make measurements as unobtrusive as possible. Observers should minimize discussions and eye contact with patients while conducting observations. Alternatively, participant observers, such as parents or older siblings, can be asked to make observations.
- Allow patients time to adapt to measurement conditions, just as a physician has a patient rest for 5 min before taking their blood pressure. This might involve disregarding information collected during the initial assessment period.

Representativeness

Obtaining representative samples of behavior is also a problem shared by all adherence measures, particularly when assessing adherence to chronic disease regimens. Regimen-related behaviors are required at specific times or opportunities and one may miss many of these opportunities to record what the person is doing. To obtain more representative samples, clinicians and researchers should

- Measure as long and often as possible (Johnson & Pennybacker, 1993).
- Use methods that are more likely to yield representative samples of behavior. For example, electronic monitors are better at this than periodic drug assays.

- Compare continuous and discontinuous methods to determine if much is lost by using the more feasible, discontinuous method. For example, one could do six structured interviews and compare the results obtained with three interviews.

Directness

A direct measure is one that measures a phenomenon in a way that captures the essence of that phenomenon. Because the focus of adherence assessment is behavior, this means directly observing behavior at the time and place of its natural occurrence (Barrios, 1988). Because this is not usually feasible, all methods for assessing adherence will vary in their degree of directness. Asking patients to report retrospectively and globally about their adherence is much more indirect than electronic monitoring or directly observing them. The issue of directness can be addressed in several ways by clinicians and researchers:

- When possible, use the most direct method available. For example, one could ask patients or family members to monitor adherence behaviors as they occur vs. asking them to rate adherence retrospectively.
- Define and refine, as needed, behavioral response classes so they are more easily understood and used by observers, including patients and families. This requires that medical providers be very specific about the nature of their recommendations. For example, vague recommendations such as, "exercise regularly" or "let your body tell you what you can do" are too vague and need some operational work.
- Compare different methods that vary in directness and empirically determine if the more indirect method converges with the more direct one (e.g., correlate pill counts with assays).

Measurement Standards

All measures of adherence vary in terms of how well they meet minimal scientific standards of measurement, including reliability, validity, and accuracy. *Reliability* refers to the consistency or reproducibility of measures (Crocker & Algina, 1986). *Validity* refers to the extent that a measure represents the phenomenon of interest or measures what it purports to measure (Anastasi, 1988). *Accuracy* (though often confused with reliability) refers to the extent that a measure reveals the "true" state of nature (Johnston & Pennypacker, 1993). The way these standards are addressed depends on the type of measure. For example, the reliability of interview measures is often tested by correlating data obtained at two points in time (test–retest reliability) while the reliability of observational measures is tested by determining agreement between two independent observers watching the same person (interobserver agreement). Accuracy is a much more difficult standard because it assumes that there is a way or an "incontrovertible" standard for judging the true state of nature (Barrios, 1988). In a very important sense, we cannot know what is "really there" because by measuring it, we change what is there. This is called the Heisenberg Uncertainty Principle in physics, where one changes the orbit of an electron when trying to measure it (Heisenberg, 1958). So what should be done? Clinicians and researchers should

- Obtain consensus among experts about the "best" measure or combination of measures for a particular type of regimen-related behavior (for example, assays plus electronic monitoring appears to be the best way to assess medication adherence). The chosen measure then becomes the "nearly incontrovertible" standard by which all measures are compared.
- Depending on the measure, obtain appropriate reliability indices, such as test–retest and internal consistency for interview measures and interobserver agreement for behavioral observations.
- Depending on the measure, obtain appropriate validity indices, such as criterion- or construct-related validity. For example, predictive validity can be demonstrated by correlating adherence with disease or health status or construct validity can be demonstrated by correlating one measure of adherence with another (more established) measure.

Interpretation or What's in a Number?

The data obtained from assessments have "no voice meaning" (Barrios, 1988). They do not speak for themselves. Data are interpreted, in part, by assigning numbers or specifying the unit of analysis. There are a number of dimensions to adherence behaviors that may be of interest, including frequency (e.g., the number of pills consumed), duration (e.g., time spent exercising), rate or the frequency per some time dimension (e.g., the frequency of exercising per week), and percent of opportunities to engage in the behavior (e.g., the percent of opportunities when PRN medications were taken when it was apparent by symptom monitoring that it was appropriate to use the medication). Since taking medications is the most common regimen-related behavior in the management of acute and chronic diseases, the following units of analysis and formulas are recommended (Kastrissios, Flowers, & Blaschke, 1996):

- *Fraction of Doses* (Fr), where, Fr = the number of doses taken ÷ the number of doses prescribed. This is the metric derived from pill counts and the product is multiplied by 100 to obtain a percentage.
- *Daily Count Index* (DCI), where DCI = the number of days on which the prescribed number of doses were taken ÷ the number of days of monitoring. Again, the product is multiplied by 100 to obtain a percentage. This can be derived from electronic monitoring but not usually pill counts (unless they are done on a daily basis, which is unlikely).

- *Prescribed Intervals Method* (PI), where PI = the number of prescribed dosing intervals (± some "forgiveness" interval, such as 2 h) ÷ the total number of possible intervals. This can be derived from electronic monitoring and the product is multiplied by 100 to obtain a percentage.
- *Exact Daily Adherence* (EAC), where EAC = the number of days when doses were taken as prescribed (including at the recommended dosing interval ± a forgiveness interval) ÷ the total number of days of monitoring. Again, this can be derived from electronic monitoring and the product is multiplied by 100 to obtain a percentage. This index is derived from the DCI and PI methods and is the most stringent of all the indices.
- *Therapeutic Coverage* (TC), where TC = the number of hours of therapeutic coverage ÷ the total number of hours monitored. Again, the product is multiplied by 100 to obtain a percentage. TC can only be approximated by electronic monitoring (with knowledge of a drug's half-life). Direct assessment of TC requires pharmacokinetic studies using assays.

Once a number is assigned to the data, clinicians and researchers have to make sense of these numbers or compare them to some standard. The ideal standard would be "biologic" or the level of adherence necessary to achieve a therapeutic response (Gordis, 1979; Haskard, DiMatteo, & Williams, 2009). Typically, however, standards have been arbitrary, such as ≥80% of medications taken as defining adequate adherence. Other approaches could include within-subject comparisons (where the patient serves as his or her own comparative yardstick) and between-subject comparisons (comparing a patient to an appropriate reference or normative group).

Clinical and Treatment Utility

Measures of adherence vary in terms of cost and feasibility for use in clinical settings. The measures that are considered more "objective," such as electronic monitoring or direct observation, are also the most expensive and the least practical for use by clinicians. Another neglected dimension of assessment is *treatment utility* or the degree to which assessments contribute to beneficial treatment outcomes (Hayes, Nelson, & Jarrett, 1987). For the most part, this has not been investigated for any of the adherence measures. For example, it is conceivable that self-monitoring by patients would demonstrate greater treatment utility than pill counts, in the sense that self-monitoring data are more likely to reveal adherence patterns and obstacles that would be useful in planning and executing interventions to improve adherence. Clinical and treatment utility issues can be addressed by

- Reducing the complexity and cost of measurement procedures to increase their clinical utility. For example, structured interviews could be simplified and tested in clinical settings.

- Improving on what clinicians already do to informally assess adherence, such as testing different approaches to questioning patients (e.g., judgmental vs. empathetic).
- Addressing treatment utility by empirically comparing different adherence measures in terms of their relative ability to produce beneficial effects, such as improved adherence and better medical outcomes. From a clinical perspective, treatment utility may be the most important dimension of assessment.

Assessing Disease and Health Outcomes

Disease and health-status parameters are initially monitored to establish a medical diagnosis. Once a diagnosis is made and a treatment plan implemented, these parameters are useful for monitoring changes in patients' status over time and informing physicians about when and how to alter the initial treatment plan. In clinical trials, outcomes are needed to demonstrate the relative efficacy of various treatments and for monitoring unintended (iatrogenic) effects of medical treatments.

Traditional medical outcomes have included clinical signs and symptoms and laboratory and diagnostic studies. For example, in asthma management, physicians are encouraged to have patients monitor their peak flow rates using a meter, record their symptoms such as coughing, and physicians are to obtain measures of lung function by spirometry in their offices or clinics (Aronson et al., 2001).

However, there is a consensus in medicine that assessment of medical outcomes needs to expand beyond traditional methods. Medical providers and researchers are beginning to appreciate that patients and their families have a unique perspective on how diseases affect important aspects of their lives, or health-related quality of life (HRQOL) (Blue & Colburn, 1996; Johnson, 1994). For example, Kaplan (1994) referred to this perspective as the "Ziggy Theorem." In one of the Ziggy cartoon strips, Ziggy asks a wise old man about the meaning of life and the wise man replies "doin stuff." Kaplan argued that the purpose of health care is to help people live longer and better and that HRQOL is defined primarily by behavioral functioning or being able to "do stuff."

Outcome assessments, particularly HRQOL measures, can help identify the psychosocial, as well as, physical consequences of chronic diseases. These can help in identifying subgroups of patient populations at risk for psychosocial adjustment problems (Spieth & Harris, 1996). They can also help evaluate the quality of medical care and inform health-care policy (Kaplan, 1994). Decisions about allocation of medical resources and services can be better made when evaluated in light of outcomes that reflect both the quantity and quality of life.

Disease and health-status indicators also need to be assessed to determine the relationship between adherence and outcome, which is either imperfect or unknown (Johnson, 1994). The whole enterprise of assessing, predicting, and improving adherence is predicated on developing reliable and valid measures of adherence and treatment outcome. HRQOL measures may be particularly useful in determining if higher adherence has positive or negative consequences for patients and their families. Measures of disease and health outcomes, such as hemoglobin A1C in diabetes, are not and should not be used as proxy measures of adherence. They need to be assessed separately and concurrently with adherence measures to determine the relationship between these two sets of variables and to determine if interventions to improve adherence also improve disease and health outcomes.

There is consensus in the literature that HRQOL is a multidimensional construct that should include at least *four core domains* (Aaronson, 1989; Palermo et al., 2008; Spieth & Harris, 1996):

- *Physical symptoms* (pain and fatigue)
- *Functional status* (ability to perform age-appropriate daily activities)
- *Psychological functioning* (affective states, adjustment indices, and self-esteem)
- *Social functioning* (the number, type, and quality of social contacts and relationships)

Another significant domain includes cognitive functioning and school-related performance (Palermo et al., 2008; Spieth & Harris, 1996). This domain is relevant for certain diseases (e.g., epilepsy) and treatments (e.g., cranial radiation) that affect the central nervous system. Also, chronically ill children and adolescents often have brief, but frequent absences from school that can adversely effect academic performance.

There have been significant advances made in the measurement of HRQOL in children and adolescents in the past decade (Eiser & Morse, 2001). There are now "well-established" generic HRQOL measures for children and adolescents (Palermo et al., 2008), such as the Child Health and Illness Profile (Starfield, Riley, & Green, 1999), the Child Health Questionnaire (Landgraf, Abetz, & Ware, 1996), the Pediatric Quality of Life Inventory (Varni, Seid, & Rode, 1999), and the Youth Quality of Life (Patrick, Edwards, & Topolski, 2002). The generic measures of HRQOL are useful in comparing HRQOL between children who have different diseases and also with healthy children. There are also a number of "well-established" disease-specific HRQOL measures (Palermo et al., 2008), such as the Child Health Assessment Questionnaire for juvenile arthritis (Singh, Athreya, Fries, & Goldsmith, 1994), the Cystic Fibrosis Questionnaire Revised (Quittner, Buu, Messer, Modi, & Watrous, 2005), the Juvenile Arthritis Functional Assessment Report (Howe et al., 1991), the Pediatric Asthma Quality of Life Questionnaire (Juniper et al., 1996), and the Pediatric Oncology Quality of Life Scale (Goodwin, Boggs, & Graham-Pole, 1994). Disease-specific HRQOL measures address unique challenges posed by specific illnesses and may have greater clinical relevance for patients and their families (Palermo et al., 2008).

Methodological Issues and Recommendations for Disease and Health Measures

Both traditional and HRQOL measures are required to conduct a comprehensive assessment of disease and health status. They are complimentary and help determine the impact of adherence to medical regimens on the physical, social, and psychological functioning of children with acute and chronic health problems. As with all measures, there are a number of methodological issues that need to be addressed.

Choice of Informants

The choice of informants varies depending on the type of disease and health-status measure chosen. Laboratory and diagnostic procedures require highly trained and skilled health-care professionals. Some traditional measures require taking a history or obtaining reports of symptoms from patients, their parents, or both. HRQOL measures are almost exclusively based on ratings obtained from patients or their parents. The perspectives of patients and their parents may differ from providers, which is the major justification for obtaining HRQOL measures. Patients may also offer different perspectives than their parents (Rosenbaum, Cadman, & Kirpalani, 1990). The term for this in the psychological assessment literature is "cross-informant variance" (Achenbach, McConaughy, & Howell, 1987). Because of this variance, reports should be obtained from multiple informants as they have unique and nonoverlapping perspectives. Clinicians and researcher should

- Utilize multiple informants including health-care providers, patients, parents, teachers, and other significant people in the lives of children to obtain a comprehensive assessment of disease and health status.
- Develop and validate traditional and HRQOL measures that can be rated by patients (Rosenbaum et al., 1990). The pediatric pain-assessment literature shows that if children are given the opportunity and a developmentally appropriate instrument, they can rate their own symptoms in a psychometrically sound way as adults (Cohen et al., 2008b; McGrath, 1990).

Representativeness

This issue concerns when and how often disease and health-status assessments are obtained. Ideally, patients would be assessed frequently enough to determine their current disease and health status and document clinically significant changes in their status from previous assessments. However, for children with chronic health problems, there are limited opportunities for obtaining measures of disease and health status, unless patients are hospitalized or seen frequently in outpatient clinics. This can create a "severity bias" in studies designed to assess the overall impact of chronic diseases. That is, patients available for assessment are those who have the most contact with the health-care system because their disease is less well controlled. The upside of this bias would be that those patients in poor disease control might also be poorly adherent and could be offered interventions to improve their adherence. Clinicians and researchers should

- Assess patients as often as possible to adequately characterize disease and health status.
- Continue to develop and validate patient and/or parental measures of disease symptoms (such as automated formats) and HRQOL, which can be completed by phone, online, or in home, school, or community settings.
- When feasible, use automated instruments to record symptoms and physiological indices, such as glucometers to record blood glucose levels and peak flow meters to record pulmonary function. Patients and their parents will need specific training and recalibration to obtain reliable and valid data for clinical and research purposes.
- The 24-h recall interview methodology for assessing adherence could be adapted to assess disease and health status. These interviews are clinically feasible as they can be done briefly by phone.

Generic vs. Disease-Specific Measures

This issue is most relevant to HRQOL measures. Both generic and disease-specific measures have their place in assessing disease and health status. Generic measures are most useful for documenting health-related disability and limitations for patients with a variety of chronic diseases. Disease-specific measures have greater clinical sensitivity and utility as they capture unique physical and psychosocial sequelae of specific diseases. Clinicians and researchers should

- Utilize both generic and disease-specific HRQOL measures, as they compliment each other and provide a more comprehensive approach to assessing outcomes.
- Although specific traditional outcome measures can be used with different patient groups (e.g., pulmonary function testing being useful for patients with asthma and CF), there is a need for a global and generic disease severity index that can be used for children and adolescents with various health problems. For example, the global severity scheme (mild intermittent, mild persistent, moderate persistent, and severe persistent) applied to patients with asthma is similar to other global severity indices (e.g., mild, moderate, and severe categories applied to patients with rheumatic diseases). Clinicians and researchers could agree on such a global rating format and develop unique criteria (based on traditional measures of disease activity) to operationalize severity categories for specific diseases.

Psychometric Standards

Measures of disease and health status must be scientific standards for reliability, validity, sensitivity, and specificity. Therefore, clinicians and researchers should

- Obtain interobserver or interrater reliability indices for measures generated by providers through direct physical examination, observation of the patient, or interpretation of laboratory and diagnostic studies. Interrater reliability of adult proxy reports of patients' symptoms and HRQOL also need to be assessed. Internal consistency reliability would be important to assess for questionnaires and rating scales that tap specific constructs or dimensions (such as functional status). Test–retest reliability may or may not be useful depending on the interval between assessments and whether the symptom or construct would be expected to be stable over a particular interval. Many symptoms of chronic disease (such as pain or fatigue) are variable or episodic and one may not expect consistency between assessment occasions.
- Obtain appropriate validity indices. Construct validity would be particularly important for HRQOL measures that seek to assess multidimensional constructs such as physical, social, and psychological functioning. Newly developed measures need to demonstrate concurrent validity with existing or standard instruments. Discriminant validity is relevant to demonstrating differences in disease and health status between healthy and ill children and among chronically ill children who are at different stages of treatment and have different disease courses.
- Ensure that traditional and HRQOL measures of disease and health status meet standards for sensitivity and specificity (Fletcher et al., 1988). This is particularly crucial for diagnostic or screening tests. Test results can be either positive or negative for the presence of a disease state, for abnormal vs. normal test results, or for different levels of disease severity. For example, an HRQOL screening instrument should correctly classify patients as having lower or higher HRQOL based on more extensive traditional or HRQOL measures.

Limiting "Physiogenic Bias"

In assessing HRQOL, investigators sometimes use a "battery" approach where a variety of psychological tests and scales are used to assess various psychosocial domains, such as affective distress and behavior problems (Spieth & Harris, 1996). These instruments were not specifically designed to assess HRQOL and they have not been normed on children and adolescents with chronic disease. Of particular concern is what has been termed "physiogenic bias" (Wells & Strickland, 1982). This means that items on psychological instruments may be tapping disease or treatment-related symptoms rather than psychological symptoms. For example, the Child Behavior Checklist (Achenbach & Rescorla, 2001) is one of the most commonly used questionnaires to document internalizing (e.g., depression) and externalizing (e.g., aggression) disorders in children with chronic disease (Lavigne & Faier-Routman, 1992). Cautions have been raised about using the Child Behavior Checklist with chronically ill children because some of the items may reflect physical rather than psychological symptoms (Perrin, Stein, & Drotar, 1991). Examples include, "stares blankly" (which may indicate seizure activity), "constipated" (which accompanies spina bifida), and "feels dizzy" (which may be a symptom of hypoglycemia). Though respondents are cautioned that these items are to be considered "physical symptoms without known medical cause," they may not be rated consistent with this caveat or the opposite pattern can occur when respondents may erroneously attribute psychological symptoms to a child's illness (Perrin et al., 1991). To minimize physiogenic bias, clinicians and researchers could

- Delete somatically loaded items, but this creates problems in scoring and interpreting standardized scales.
- Make sure that respondents understand that they are being asked to rate symptoms that do not relate to disease or treatment-related symptoms.
- Develop separate norms for children and adolescents with various chronic diseases.
- Conduct studies to assess whether physiogenic bias affects standardized measures of psychological functioning for children and adolescents with chronic illness. This has been done with chronically ill adults and would be an important contribution to the pediatric literature.

Clinical Feasibility, Utility, and Relevance

Measures of disease and health status may be reliable, valid, and yield clinically useful information but may be underutilized because they are not feasible. Clinical feasibility, utility, and relevance can be enhanced by

- Making instruments and scales understandable and easy to use for providers, patients, and parents. Because there is a limited amount of time during routine clinic visits, instruments should not overburden respondents or assessors. In outpatient subspecialty clinics, routine follow-up visits are often limited to 15 min or less and priority is given to essential and traditional measures of disease activity (e.g., physical examination and laboratory tests). This means that administration time for HRQOL measures needs to be 10 min or less. Unfortunately, most HRQOL measures do not meet this standard. Research is needed to shorten and revalidate current HRQOL measures.
- Specifying a time interval (e.g., the past week) when asking patients or proxies about symptoms and HRQOL dimensions. The time interval should be short enough to limit distortion and bias due to memory, which usually means over the past month or less.

- Providing patients or proxies a comparative reference point for symptom and HRQOL ratings, such as how they are functioning compared to before diagnosis, treatment, or since their last visit (Aaronson, 1989).
- Allowing patients or proxies to assess the importance, as well as the severity of problems in various HRQOL domains (Gill & Feinstein, 1994). For example, chronic illness may limit children's participation in organized sports, but depending on their pre-illness history this dimension may or may not be important to a particular child.
- Augmenting standard or supplied items on HRQOL instruments with open-ended supplemental items that allow patients or proxies to add unique opinions and reactions. In short, clinicians need to give patients and their parents the opportunity to communicate information they did not think to ask about.

Conclusions

Much work still needs to be done to develop reliable, valid, accurate, and clinically useful measures of adherence, disease status, and HRQOL. Health-care professionals need all of these measures to show that interventions that enhance adherence also result in improvements in disease outcomes and HRQOL. A critical issue is the developmental level, particularly cognitive maturity, of children asked to report on adherence and their disease and health status. The self-report measures in Table 4.2 have generally not been validated for use with children less than 8 years of age. Parent proxy adherence measures may be more appropriate for younger children, but more research is needed to determine if younger children can reliably rate their own adherence. The same is true for self-report measures of disease, health status, and HRQOL. For example, pain has been reliably and validly rated by children as young as 3 years of age, if they are given an age-appropriate measure (Stinson, Kavanagh, Yamada, Gill, & Stevens, 2006). HRQOL measures, such as the PedsQL, have been completed by children as young as 5 years of age and for those younger than 5, parent proxy measures are available for children as young as 2 years of age (Varni et al., 1999). However, we must be careful not to use age as a proxy measure of cognitive maturity, but directly assess whether children understand and can use measures we have developed.

Another issue relevant to adherence and disease/health-status measures is establishing standards for "meaningful or clinically significant improvement" on the measures we develop.

As stated before, the ideal standard for adherence measures would be "biologic" or the level of adherence necessary to achieve a therapeutic response (Gordis, 1979). For example, if the adherence rate to antiretroviral medications needs to be $\geq 95\%$ to achieve a significant reduction in viral load, then our interventions which help patients achieve this standard would produce clinically significant results. Standards would also need to be established for disease/health status and HRQOL measures. For example, with a generic HRQOL, would the standard be that we help patients achieve a level of HRQOL that is in the average range of scores (plus or minus one standard deviation) for appropriate normative groups of healthy children and adolescents? For self-report measures of pain, a 30% reduction in the rating of pain intensity has been suggested for defining clinically significant improvement on this symptom (Rowbothan, 2001). As standards evolve, we will be able to demonstrate to patients, families, health-care providers, politicians, and insurance carriers that our adherence interventions produce clinically meaningful improvements in the lives of chronically ill children and adolescents.

Chapter 5
Strategies for Improving Adherence to Pediatric Medical Regimens

Adherence-improvement strategies can be broadly classified as *educational, orga-nizational*, and *behavioral* (Dunbar, Marshall, & Hovell, 1979). *Educational strategies* primarily rely on verbal, written, computer-based, or Web-based information designed to enlighten patients and their families about diseases, treatment regimens, potential negative side effects of treatment, and the importance of consistent adherence. *Organizational strategies* target ways in which health care is delivered, including increasing access to health-care services, simplifying regimens, and increasing provider supervision of regimens. *Behavioral strategies* refer to behavior-change techniques to alter specific adherence behaviors such as patient and parental monitoring of regimens, problem-solving, contracting, and token reinforcement programs.

Before describing these strategies, an important caveat is in order. *Efforts to alter adherence to medical regimens should only be considered when there is good evidence that adherence problems are compromising the health and well-being of the patient.* The corollary of this is *if a patient is doing well, then leave well-enough alone.*

The purpose of this chapter is to describe (1) educational strategies for improving adherence to pediatric medical regimens, including the goals, content, and methods of education; (2) organizational strategies for improving adherence to pediatric medical regimens, including reducing the complexity and negative side effects of regimens, increasing provider supervision, and improving provider–patient communication and relationships; (3) specific behavior-change strategies for improving adherence to pediatric medical regimens, including monitoring, prompting, reinforcement, and discipline techniques; (4) using barriers assessments or a functional analysis approach to individualize adherence interventions; and (5) technology-based approaches to educating families and promoting adherence.

M.A. Rapoff, *Adherence to Pediatric Medical Regimens*, Issues in Clinical Child Psychology, DOI 10.1007/978-1-4419-0570-3_5,
© Springer Science+Business Media, LLC 2010

Educational Strategies for Improving Adherence

The "Why?" or Goals of Education

Clinicians need to be clear about why they educate. The overall goal of education is to increase patient and family knowledge about diseases, treatments, and the importance of consistent adherence. In short, clinicians want patients and their families to "know" stuff. The British philosopher Gilbert Ryle made an important distinction between two types of "knowing": *knowing that* and *knowing how* (Ryle, 1949). *Knowing that* means patients and their families are able to convey in verbal and/or written form that they understand information presented to them. Providers often ask patients and families or give them questionnaires to determine if they know about diseases, treatments that have been prescribed, and the rationale for such treatments. For example, providers would want a patient with type 1 diabetes (among other things) to describe how diabetes involves failure of her pancreas to produce insulin, how she should check her blood glucose and perform insulin injections, and the importance of adjusting insulin doses based on diet, blood glucose levels, exercise, and stress. The patient may demonstrate that she "knows" this information by responding correctly to verbal or written questions and prompts. However, an additional type of "knowing" is essential. *Knowing how* means patients and families are able to actually do something according to some specific standards. Referring to the patient with diabetes, providers would want some behavioral evidence that she can correctly test her blood glucose and properly prepare, time, and inject insulin based on her specific dietary, blood glucose, exercise, and stress levels. Providers need to make sure that patients and their families have a specific knowledge base relative to diseases and treatments and the necessary behavioral repertoire to carry out prescribed regimens.

The "What?" or Specific Objectives and Content of Education

Educational content and objectives are determined by the type of disease and recommended treatments. For acute conditions, such as otitis media, the treatment is relatively straightforward in that patients are required to take antibiotic medications over relatively short periods of time (5–14 days). The situation is more complex for chronic conditions as patients have to adhere to multiple regimen tasks, such as taking medications, following special diets, doing general and/or specific exercises, and monitoring symptoms.

The provider who prescribes a particular regimen is responsible for determining the specific treatment plan based on the empirical literature and resulting consensus practice guidelines. Once a specific treatment plan has been developed, patients and families would generally need to receive the following core information (JRA is used here as an example):

What the patient has. Information needs to be given about the disease, including its diagnostic label (e.g., JRA), possible causes (e.g., unknown, but autoimmunity implicated along with some viral or other type of trigger), course (e.g., the subtype of JRA determines the extent and severity of joint involvement and associated symptoms), and prognosis (e.g., with most children, JRA is controlled, but not cured and the prognosis for a normal and functional lifespan is generally good).

What needs to be done to control the disease. Patients and families need to know what they are to do (e.g., take anti-inflammatory medications, do special exercises, and wear protective splints on involved joints at night) and why (e.g., to reduce joint inflammation, control pain, increase joint range of motion, and avoid joint deformities).

Potential negative side effects of treatment and how to reduce these. A list of possible side effects should be given and how likely they are to be experienced (e.g., gastrointestinal irritation with medications for treating JRA are common). Also, specific ways to reduce side effects should be suggested (e.g., take medications with food to reduce irritation or warm affected joints before exercising by doing exercises in a hot tub).

The benefits of consistent adherence and strategies for enhancing adherence. Patients and their families need to be informed about how consistent adherence could be beneficial (e.g., following JRA treatment recommendations consistently can reduce inflammation and pain, increase functional activities, and reduce the need for additional diagnostic and treatment procedures). The strategies discussed in this chapter can be described verbally and in written form to patients and families (e.g., how to monitor, prompt, and reinforce children's adherence to treatment recommendations). For example, I wrote a booklet for parents of children with rheumatic diseases which describes ways they can help their children be more consistent in following treatment recommendations (Rapoff, 1997).

The "How?" of Educational Strategies

How patients and families are educated is critical and is often inadequate or infrequent. A number of general principles and strategies can be recommended:

Education as an ongoing process. Particularly with chronic diseases, patient and family education is not accomplished in a single session when patients are newly diagnosed. Patients and their families are often distressed when a chronic condition is first diagnosed, and this distress may interfere with retention of information about the condition and its treatment. Also, chronic conditions are complex and have a variable course, which necessitates modifications in treatment plans and the need to re-educate. Thus, education continues over time and involves repetition and rewording of information as needed.

Effective Verbal Communication. Verbal instructions to patients and families must be clear, concise, and relevant to educational objectives. To facilitate patient or parent understanding and recall of information presented, clinicians should

- Be friendly rather than businesslike.
- Provide instructions clearly and concisely and early in the presentation.

- Stress the importance of the instructions.
- Use short words and sentences, avoiding jargon.
- Use explicit categorization (e.g., "I am going to tell you what is wrong, what tests need to be done, and how to treat your child's illness.").
- Repeat information as needed, particularly when children are first diagnosed as patients and parents may experience emotional distress which interferes with recall.
- Check for understanding of the information and openly encourage questions, including any barriers to adherence anticipated by the patient or family.
- Determine if patient and family expectations and/or concerns have been addressed and secure a verbal commitment to attempt to follow the prescribed regimen.

Written Communication and Other Media. Clinicians should use written materials (pamphlets, brochures, or instruction sheets) and other media (videos, computer programs, and Web sites) to reinforce and enhance verbal instructions. However, most clinicians are not well trained in how to develop these educational materials. This situation often results in health education reading material that exceeds the reading level of parents and children (Singh, 1995). For example, one study found that reading grade level of written asthma plans ranged from 4.9 to 9.2, although the recommended level is fifth grade or lower (Forbis & Aligne, 2002). This situation is more complex for patients. Written and other educational materials must be designed to address normal developmental variations in cognitive development for children at various ages.

In the case of written material, readability is one critical dimension. There are a number of formulas for calculating readability, including Dale-Chall, Fry, Flesch, and SMOG (Meade & Smith, 1991). These formulas consider the average number of syllables per word, average number of words per sentence, and/or word length in characters to calculate a standard reading score or approximate reading grade level from samples of a text. There are specific computer programs (Meade & Smith, 1991) and options within word-processing programs that will rapidly calculate different readability formulas. However, there are variables, other than readability level, which should be considered in developing educational materials. These are summarized in Table 5.1.

Clinicians may not need to develop educational materials from scratch. There are well-developed educational materials available for patients with a variety of chronic health problems and their families. Also, national organizations provide pamphlets and information on Web sites for patients and their families (for example, see Oermann, Gerich, Ostosh, & Zaleski, 2003 for their recommendations for the top 10 best Web sites for asthma education). Clinicians need to carefully review generic educational materials to determine their appropriateness for their specific population of patients and families. Also, families need to be cautioned that not all information available on Web sites is correct. They should access Web sites sanctioned by governmental agencies (e.g., Maternal and Child Health, NIH) or national foundations with professional oversight (e.g., the Arthritis Foundation).

Table 5.1 Factors to consider when developing health education materials

Factor	Recommendations
Organization	Use abstracts, headings, subheadings, and questions at the beginning, end, and/or interspersed throughout the text. Make sure paragraphs/sections address a single purpose or idea.
Writing style	Use active rather than passive voice (e.g., "take this medicine right after breakfast" rather than "this medicine should be taken after breakfast")
Illustrations	Use pictures, drawings, diagrams, tables, graphs, or charts to illustrate concepts and summarize material. Make sure these are relevant to the content of the text and appropriate for the target audience.
Typography	Use legibly and attractive type fonts, sizes, formats, and colors.
Tailoring	Tailor material to target audience. Consider age, gender, cultural and experiential factors, and attention level. Use "focus groups" or small groups of persons from the intended audience to preview material and make changes prior to final version.
Health literacy	Patients and families need to listen, read, understand, and use health information appropriately. Readability level generally should be at the 5th grade and lower for adults and matched to the reading level of children.

Source: Adapted from recommendations by Forbis and Aligne (2002), Meade and Smith (1991), and Singh (1995).

They can also read articles that have reviewed and evaluated the content of Web sites (Croft & Peterson, 2002; Oermann et al., 2003).

There is good evidence that educational approaches combined with behavioral strategies are effective in improving adherence to regimens for acute diseases (Rapoff & Christophersen, 1982; Wu & Roberts, 2008). When patients are diagnosed with an acute illness, such as otitis media, a standard written handout can be given to parents. Drug companies often supply these types of handouts, along with calendars or other types of monitoring forms to help patients and/or parents keep track of medication doses. Other strategies need to be added for more complex, chronic disease regimens.

Modeling and Behavioral Rehearsal. Clinicians need to be certain that patients and their families know how to carry out regimen tasks. It is often not sufficient to provide verbal and written instructions, particularly for complex regimens. The clinician needs to model how to execute more complex regimen tasks, give the patient and parent opportunities to practice the tasks, and provide corrective feedback as needed. For example, children with asthma often have difficulty with proper administration of inhaled medications using a metered-dose inhaler (MDI). This is critical as improper use of an MDI will result in medication being deposited into the mouth or throat and not into the lungs. Patients and their parents can be provided with specific written instructions with illustrations (see Fig. 5.1). However, in most cases, proper MDI technique will need to be modeled by the clinician and patients or parents will need opportunities to practice and receive corrective feedback from the clinician.

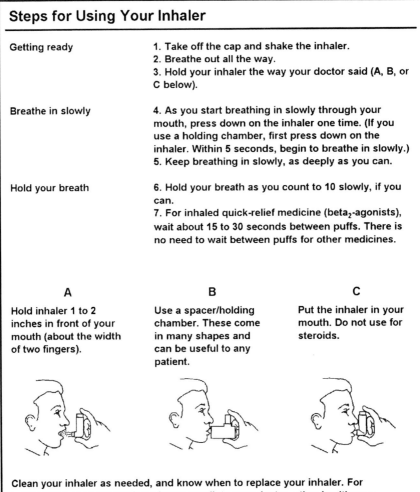

Steps for Using Your Inhaler

Getting ready	1. Take off the cap and shake the inhaler. 2. Breathe out all the way. 3. Hold your inhaler the way your doctor said (A, B, or C below).
Breathe in slowly	4. As you start breathing in slowly through your mouth, press down on the inhaler one time. (If you use a holding chamber, first press down on the inhaler. Within 5 seconds, begin to breathe in slowly.) 5. Keep breathing in slowly, as deeply as you can.
Hold your breath	6. Hold your breath as you count to 10 slowly, if you can. 7. For inhaled quick-relief medicine (beta$_2$-agonists), wait about 15 to 30 seconds between puffs. There is no need to wait between puffs for other medicines.

A	B	C
Hold inhaler 1 to 2 inches in front of your mouth (about the width of two fingers).	Use a spacer/holding chamber. These come in many shapes and can be useful to any patient.	Put the inhaler in your mouth. Do not use for steroids.

Clean your inhaler as needed, and know when to replace your inhaler. For instructions, read the package insert or talk to your doctor, other health care provider, or pharmacist.

Fig. 5.1 Instructions for using a metered-dose inhaler. Adapted from National Asthma Education and Prevention Program (1997). In the public domain

Summary of Educational Strategies

Clinicians need to take seriously their role as educators. Patients and their families deserve to receive high-quality education that fosters knowledge about diseases and their treatments and the necessary behavioral skills for being able to carry out regimens. Clinicians should remember that the desired outcome of educational efforts is to affect behavior change and not just improve scores on standard tests of knowledge. Also, there is good evidence that educational strategies are *necessary but not sufficient* to sustain adherence, particularly to complex chronic disease regimens (Rapoff, 1999). Other strategies will often be needed.

Organizational Strategies for Improving Adherence

Increasing Accessibility to Health Care

Some patients do not regularly contact the health-care system. Accessibility to health care can be limited because of financial reasons, transportation problems, and inconveniences inherent to health-care settings. Accessibility can be increased by putting patients and their families in contact with social service agencies that can assist them in finding transportation and medical coverage. Also, health care can be brought to the patient through outreach clinics in schools, churches, or even in the patient's home. These types of outreach clinics may be cost-effective, if they reduce morbidity, mortality, and overuse of expensive medical services, such as emergency room visits.

Consumer-Friendly Clinical Settings

Consider the following scenario. A mother brings her sick child to an outpatient acute care clinic, where she is confronted with harried and terse personnel who take 30 minutes to check her child in to see a doctor. She takes her child to the waiting room, which is full of other parents with sick and crying children. The waiting area is sparse, devoid of proper play materials for children. After waiting another 15–30 min (by which time her child is quite irritable and crying), she is then ushered into a clinic room, which is sparse and devoid of any books or play materials for her child. Her child is finally seen by a staff doctor or resident, after seeing a nurse and medical student. Her child has been never seen by this doctor before and so the mother has to catch the doctor up on her child's relevant medical history. She is briefly told what is wrong with her child and given a prescription, with little time to ask questions or receive assurance that her child is not gravely ill. Sound familiar? This scenario may be embellished, but something like this can be observed in teaching hospital clinics around the country. This hypothetical mother may likely leave this clinic in no mood to cooperate or return to the clinic any time soon, unless her child continues to be acutely ill, in which case she may elect to take her child to the emergency room. The message here is that clinical settings need to be consumer-friendly.

A consumer-friendly setting would yield a very different scenario. Pleasant and helpful personnel would greet the mother and child, and the child would be checked into the clinic in a timely fashion. The waiting area would be full of a variety of interesting and developmental appropriate play materials. There may even be volunteers who would play with and read to children. The child would only stay in the waiting area for 10–15 min and then be escorted to a clinic room, that again has appropriate play and reading materials. A doctor, very familiar to the mother and child, would then enter the room, sometimes accompanied by a medical student. After the child was examined, the mother would be given a thorough explanation of what is wrong with her child and what the doctor is recommending to treat her child's illness. The mother would also be given ample opportunity to have her questions and concerns addressed. She would then leave the clinic with specific and understandable instructions on how to treat her child and what to do if her child is not better after a specified period of time. The mother in this consumer-friendly scenario is likely to leave this clinic more satisfied and more favorably inclined to carry out the doctor's treatment recommendations.

Perhaps providers would do well to consider health care as a competitive business (in the good sense of this) where they have to outdo their competitors in delivering the best and most satisfying service to their customers. Taking this position would most likely result in having more attractive and responsive clinical settings. There would also be continuity of care, where the same physician sees a child at each clinic visit. This is likely to enhance patient and family satisfaction and improve adherence. Continuity of care would also reduce the likelihood of conflicting and incongruent advice being offered which can occur when different providers are involved with the same child.

Increasing Provider Supervision

Provider supervision can take many forms. The most basic form is asking about adherence-related issues during clinic visits. This needs to be done in a nonjudgmental and specific way, which is more likely to foster open communication and effective problem solving. If the patient and family have agreed to follow a particular regimen and still experience difficulty with being consistent, the provider can ask: "What gets in the way or keeps you from being consistent?" This type of questioning can lead to effective problem solving about how to reduce identified barriers.

Providers can increase supervision of regimens in other ways. Patients can be brought back to clinic for more frequent follow-up visits. This allows for more opportunities to monitor progress and address any problems. Also, patients and families can phone a "report line" or phone number staffed during the day and recorded after hours by an answering machine. Staff can then respond quickly to parental or patient concerns and address barriers to adherence (Rapoff & Barnard, 1991). Clinic personnel could also call patients and families at critical times when adherence is likely to be a problem. For example, many patients do not continue with 10-day courses of antibiotics after the 4th or 5th day. Clinic personnel could phone parents to remind them to give antibiotics to their children for the full 10 or 14 days to eradicate infections.

In order to properly monitor regimen adherence, providers need to remember what they prescribed. Sometimes there is confusion between patients and providers about what has been prescribed. This most often occurs with chronic disease regimens when multiple regimen components have been prescribed. To minimize confusion, providers, patients, or parents can keep track of regimen requirements and changes, which are made over time, using a standard form (see Fig. 5.2 for a sample form for patients with cystic fibrosis).

Simplifying and Minimizing Negative Side Effects of Regimens

Patients and their families have a finite amount of time, energy, and resources to devote to medical regimens, if they are to maintain some semblance of a normal

Prescribed Treatment Plan – Cystic Fibrosis

[Every Question Must be Answered *Even If Not Prescribed!*]

Today's Date: _____ Patient Name _____ Dr._____

Please Circle, Check Off or Fill In the Correct Response

1. AIRWAY CLEARANCE: *Not Prescribed*

Primary: CPT Flutter Acapella Vest PEP device Exercise Other:_____

Frequency: PRN (As needed) 1X/day 2X/day 3X/day 4X/day Other:_____

Duration: 6-10 min 11-15 min 16-20 min 21-25 min 26+ min

Secondary: CPT Flutter Acapella Vest PEP device Exercise Other:_____

Frequency: PRN 1X/day 2X/day 3X/day Duration: 6-10 min 11-15 min 16-20 min 21-25 min 26+ min

2. MEDICATIONS:

Oral Steroids: *Not Prescribed* Prednisone _____ mg Other:_____

Frequency: ____day taper OR # of pills ____/ 1x/day 2x/day 3x/day 4x/day Duration:_____

Oral Non-steroidal Anti-Inflamatory Agent: *Not Prescribed* Ibuprofen____ mg Other:_____ ____mg

Frequency: 1X/day 2X/day 3X/day 4X/day

Leukotriene Modifiers : *Not prescribed* Accolate Singulair Dosage: ____mg 1x/pm

Oral Antibiotics: *Not Prescribed* Cipro Levaquin Augmentin Zithromax Ceclor Amoxicillin

Biaxin Septra Keflex Other:_____ ____/mg

Frequency: 1X/day 2X/day 3X/day 4X/day 5X/day 6X/day Duration: 10 days 14 days 28 days

Vitamins: ADEK liquid ____ml OR # of tabs____ Frequency: 1X/day 2X/day 3X/day

Vitamin K ____mg Frequency: 1X/day 2X/day 3X/day

Vitamin E ____I.U. Frequency: 1X/day 2X/day 3X/day

Other:_____ Frequency: 1X/day 2X/day 3X/day

Digestive: Zantac ____mg Protonic ___mg Actigall/Urso ___mg Prevacid____mg Prilosec____mg Other____

Frequency: PRN (As needed) 1X/day 2X/day 3X/day 4X/day 5X/day 6X/day

Fig. 5.2 A written treatment plan for cystic fibrosis. Reprinted by permission from Dr. Alexander Quittner

Patient Name:_____   Date:_____

Allergies/Antihistamines:

Claritin ___mg   Zyrtec _____mg   Allegra___mg   <u>Frequency:</u>   PRN (As needed) 1X/day 2X/day 3X/day

Flonase, Rhinocort. Nasonex ____/sprays   <u>Frequency:</u>   PRN (As needed) 1X/day 2X/day 3X/day

Other:_____   <u>Frequency:</u>   PRN (As needed) 1X/day 2X/day 3X/day

3. NEBULIZED TREATMENTS:

Medications/Dose: Albuterol _____   Saline _____   Other: _____

    <u>Frequency:</u>   *Not Prescribed*   *PRN (As needed)*   1X/day   2X/day   3X/day   4X/day

Pulmozyme: *Not Prescribed*   1X/day   2X/day   <u>Duration:</u> _____

Inhaled Antibiotics: *Not Prescribed*   Gentamicin   Colistin   Other: _____   _____mg

    <u>Frequency:</u>   1X/day   2X/day   3X/day   4X/day   <u>Duration:</u> _____

    TOBI: *Not Prescribed*   PRN (As needed)   28-day cycle: on ____/off ____   1X/day   2X/day   Duration:_____

4. METERED DOSE INHALERS:

Bronchodilator: *Not Prescribed*   Albuterol   Pirbuterol   Terbutaline   Salmeterol   Other: _____

    <u>Frequency:</u>   PRN (As needed)   1X/day   2X/day   3X/day   4X/day   # of puffs/treatment: _____

Inhaled Anti-Inflammatory Agents: Steroidal:

    Not Prescribed   Pulmacort   Flovent – 44/110/220   Beclomethasone (Beclovent/Vanceril)   Other: _____

    <u>Frequency:</u>   PRN (As needed)   1X/day   2X/day   3X/day   4X/day   # of puffs/treatment: _____

    Combination Inhaler: *Not prescribed*   Advair   Dose: 100/50   250/50   500/50   **Frequency:**   1 inhalation 2x/day

5. ENZYMES: *Not Prescribed*

Type: Creon # ___ (e.g. 5)   Ultrase # ___ (e.g. MT6)   # ___   Pancrease # ___ (e.g. MT4)   Other: _____

Dose per meal:	1	2	3	4	5	6	7	8	9	10	11	12
Dose per snack:	1	2	3	4	5	6	7	8	9	10	11	12
Dose per tube feed:	1	2	3	4	5	6	7	8	9	10	11	12

6. NUTRITIONAL SUPPLEMENTS: *Not Prescribed*   Boost   Scandishake   Ensure   Pediasure   Other: _____

    <u>Frequency:</u>   1X/day 2X/day 3X/day 4X/day 5X/day 6X/day

7. TUBE FEEDINGS: *Not Prescribed*   Deliver Pediasure   Peptamen   Other: _____

    Feeding Schedule: _____ (e.g. overnight drip ____ rate/hour)

8. BOOSTING CALORIES: *Not Prescribed*   Increase intake at meals   Add snack(s)   Additional meals

Other: _____

Patient Name:_____   Date:_____

9. OTHER INSTRUCTIONS: _____

<u>Physician:</u>   (last names of all clinic physicians are listed here to be circled)

Date of NEXT visit: _____

Fig. 5.2   (continued)

family life (Patterson, 1985). Providers need to help them strike this balance by minimizing the complexity, costs, and negative side effects of regimens (Winnick, Lucas, Hartman, & Toll, 2005).

Reducing complexity might involve prescribing once-daily vs. multiple daily dosing of antibiotics for shorter periods of time (5 days vs. 10–14 days). Also, multicomponent regimens can sometimes be introduced in a gradual and step-by-step fashion. The complexity is then increased as the patient masters prior steps in a sequence of components ordered in terms of difficulty level. For example, exercise programs for chronically ill children could be limited to short periods and then gradually increased as the patient demonstrates mastery and increased stamina.

Tailoring regimens to patients' lifestyles and schedules can also reduce the demands of regimens. Clinicians can assess typical daily schedules of patients to determine how the prescribed regimen can be integrated into the patients' daily routines. It is usually easier to alter regimens than to alter established patient routines. To do this requires asking a patient and her family about a "typical day," where the clinician obtains information about what the child does from the time she wakes up until she goes to bed. The clinician then negotiates with the patient and family about how to integrate regimen requirements into the daily routine and manage any anticipated problems (e.g., what to do when you are away from home and have to take medications). My colleagues and I worked with one child with JRA who disliked doing specific exercises, but she enjoyed watching afternoon cartoons following school. We worked out a plan with the patient and her parents that allowed her do exercises while watching cartoons (an innovation added by her mother was to briefly turn off the TV if she stopped exercising).

With medications, parents may prefer oral liquid medications as they are easier to administer to younger children (Winnick et al., 2005). A surprising number of children and adolescents (and even adults) find it difficult to swallow pills, particularly larger ones. One retrospective chart review of 23 patients with HIV (4–21 years) who had received pill-swallowing training found that they experienced a significant improvement in adherence and related improvements in viral load (Garvie, Lensing, & Rai, 2007). A pill-swallowing protocol that has been in used for a variety of chronic diseases can be found in Table 5.2.

Patients sometimes stop regimens because they experience negative side effects. Providers need to help patients anticipate and minimize side effects as much as possible. Some medications, such as antibiotics or nonsteroidal anti-inflammatory drugs, cause gastrointestinal irritation and pain, which can be reduced by taking medications with food or taking antacids. Exercise can also be painful, for anyone, but particularly for children with rheumatic diseases. Gradually increasing the intensity of exercise or exercising in a hot tub can minimize discomfort.

Summary of Organizational Strategies

Clinicians should avoid the tendency to assign "blame" to patients and their families for adherence problems. Clinicians might well look "inward" first, to determine

Tables 5.2 Pill-swallowing protocol used for children with cystic fibrosis

Encouraging pill swallowing in children

A behavioral intervention

Why is pill swallowing important?

Difficulty swallowing pills is a significant barrier to adherence in children. Learning to swallow pills is important for children who must regularly take oral medications. Swallowing pills without difficulty increases adherence, convenience for parents, and the efficacy of medications.

Behavioral Intervention

o Uses successive approximations (steps) to establish the behavior (swallowing pills)
o Positive reinforcement (rewards) help to get the behavior going and maintained

Preparation

o Create a pill-swallowing kit including candy (sprinkles, mini M&Ms, Nerds), small cups for water, empty gel capsules, stickers, sticker charts.
o Ask parents to save gel capsules when they remove enzyme beads; these capsules can be used later. Or they can purchase gel capsules over the Internet.

Assessment

Get approval from the child's physician; check for allergies to the candies
o Ask parents if eating candy is okay

Instructions for successive approximations

Step 1: Ask the child to swallow a sip of water. Praise the child, "great job swallowing the water!" Let the child pick another sticker for this first success!
Step 2: Start with the smallest candy (sprinkles). Let the child feel the candy on their tongue and melting down their throat.
Step 3: Ask the child to "place the candy on the middle of your tongue. Tilt your head back a little, take a drink of water, and swallow the 'pill'."
Step 4: If the child is comfortable with Steps 1–3, go on to the next larger candy.

Hierarchy

After several consecutive successes, the child may move on to the next size candy "pill." You can set the pace for moving through the hierarchy below:
o Sprinkles
o Mini M&Ms
o Nerds
o Empty pill gel capsule
o Finally, take the prescribed pill!

First session

o Praise the child for both effort and success.
o Most children find swallowing these sprinkles surprisingly easy.
o Sessions generally last 5–10 min and should be fun!
o Length of the session should be based on the child's attention and skill.

Tables 5.2 (continued)

Encouraging pill swallowing in children

---

o If the child has difficulty with a larger piece of candy, end the session with a success by having the child swallow a smaller piece.

o {You can move backwards on the hierarchy at any time!}

Homework

o Give the parent samples of each candy, blank sticker charts, and stickers to continue the program at home.

o Encourage the parent to practice each day and to reinforce progress with praise and stickers.

o Be specific about when they will practice (e.g., before dinner).

o After the child earns a certain number of stickers (determined by the parent), the child can earn a small prize, such as crayons, a coloring book, or extra time playing video games or with parents.

o Check progress and continue the pill-swallowing program at the next clinic visit.

o This can also be done if child is in hospital.

Future sessions

o Begin the next session with the size candy the child swallowed at the end of the previous session.

o Once the child progresses through the 3 types of candy, he/she can swallow the empty pill gel capsule.

o Some children move through the hierarchy easily in one or two sessions. Other children may require 2–6 sessions.

o Be patient and make it fun!

o Continue to praise and reinforce pill swallowing until the behavior is well established.

Other strategies at home

o Put the pill into a spoonful of ice cream, applesauce, or pudding and let it slide down your child's throat.

o Swallow the pill with milk or juice instead of water to change the thickness and taste of the liquid.

Source: Adapted with permission from a handout by Alexandra L. Quittner, Ph.D., Kristen K. Marciel, Ph.D., Avani C. Modi, Ph.D., & Ivette Cruz, M.S., *supported by NIH grant #RO1 HL69736*.

what they do or fail to do that makes it more difficult for patients to follow prescribed medical regimens. Patients and families are burdened enough with the normal daily challenges of life plus additional problems created by disease and treatments. This burden can be lessened by reducing the complexity, costs, and aversive aspects of regimens.

Behavioral Strategies for Improving Adherence

Parental Monitoring and Supervision

The lack of parental monitoring and supervision of medical treatments is a significant contributor to nonadherence, particularly to chronic disease regimens. This becomes critical as patients move into adolescence, where parental monitoring is episodic or nonexistent. Parents of teenagers can appreciate the conflict of trying to be sensitive to their teenager's need for autonomy while recognizing the necessity of providing continued monitoring and guidance. Clinicians need to emphasize to parents not to abruptly or completely discontinuing monitoring and support of their children, even during adolescence.

In cooperation with their children, parents can monitor adherence to treatments using standard forms, such as the one shown in Fig. 5.3. These forms can be placed on the refrigerator and parents and children can "check off" when a particular regimen task has been completed. This type of monitoring may be used on a daily basis until adherence is consistently high, then faded out, and reinstated if adherence

TREATMENT REGIMEN MONITORING CHART

Name _____   Dates _____

Regimen Requirement	Sun	Mon	Tues	Wed	Thurs	Fri	Sat
Medications							
Exercises							
Diet							
Other							

Fig. 5.3 An example of a regimen-monitoring form

drops. Parents can also check medication supplies (e.g., pill containers or inhalers) and devices (e.g., blood glucose meters) for indirect evidence that their children are adherent or nonadherent.

Supervision of regimens needs to be done in a way that is sensitive to the developmental capabilities of children. With younger children, parents will likely have primary responsibility for administering treatments and monitoring disease symptoms. Supervision can then be reduced (but never completely discontinued) as children demonstrate that they can administer their treatments and monitor their disease symptoms consistently.

To avoid unnecessary conflict, parents should be cautioned to monitor and supervise regimens in a sympathetic and constructive way. They can sympathize (e.g., "I understand that it's hard to remember to take your medicine.") but also communicate to their children the importance of adherence and that they are available to help their children be consistent (e.g., "It's very important that you remember to take your medicine. Let's think of how we can help you to remember.").

Prompting Adherence

During a conversation with an 11-year-old boy with JRA who had been referred to me for nonadherence to medications, I asked him what prevented him from being consistent in taking his medications. He said, "It doesn't remind me." Sometimes patients forget or their symptoms are apparently not salient enough to prompt adherence. In these situations, salient and reliable prompts are needed to promote adherence. This can be done in several ways. Monitoring adherence and pairing regimen tasks with regularly occurring events (e.g., taking medications with meals) may help to prompt adherence (Park & Kidder, 1996). Also, relatively inexpensive watches or pill containers are available, which can be programmed to beep at multiple times during the day to prompt adherence. Hand-held PDA programs can also be programmed to give audile and text reminders for taking medications or doing other regimen requirements (see the On-Time Rx® PDA program at www.AmeliaPlex.com, accessed on November 26, 2008).

Adherence Incentives

Ideally, patients are prescribed effective treatments that rapidly and pervasively resolve or control their health problems. Thus, the incentive to adhere is that patients get better, feel better, and do better. However, this ideal situation is not consistent with the experience of most patients, families, and providers. For example, nonsteroidal anti-inflammatory medications in the treatment of JRA may not effectively control symptoms for at least 8 weeks from the initiation of therapy (Lovell et al., 1984). More immediate incentives or positive consequences need to be programmed to bridge the temporal gap between initial adherence and the more long-range benefits of adherence. If adherence is then sustained, maximal therapeutic effects may be obtained and provide "natural" consequences (in the form of improved health and function) to further maintain adherence.

My colleagues and I have taken this approach in utilizing token reinforcement and other programmed positive consequences to improve and sustain adherence to regimens for JRA (Pieper et al., 1989; Rapoff et al., 1984; Rapoff et al., 1988a, 1988b) and asthma (da Costa, Rapoff, Lemanek, & Goldstein, 1997). The basic format has been similar. We worked with families to identify target adherence behaviors to operationalize, measure, and alter. The reinforcement program involves giving tokens (points or chips) for adherence, taking away tokens for nonadherence, and requiring the patient to purchase basic and special privileges with the tokens. Once such program, the Exchange Program, is reproduced in Fig. 5.4. These types of programs have been particularly effective in improving adherence to chronic disease regimens.

Another frequently used strategy, particularly with adolescents, is contracting. Patients and their parents are taught basic communication and negotiation skills.

THE EXCHANGE PROGRAM FOR IMPROVING MEDICATION ADHERENCE

The Exchange Program is a way for you to encourage your child to take his/her medications more consistently. It is based on the well-established principle that people tend to engage in behaviors that bring rewards and/or allows them to avoid unpleasant events. In order to earn basic privileges, your child will be required to take all his/her medications in front of you each day. Your child can also earn special privileges (usually engaged in on the weekend) by earning basics on a certain number of days per week. "Basic" and "special" privileges are described below with specific examples.

In addition to awarding privileges, it is very important to praise your child immediately after he/she takes his/her medications. In the long run, the positive attention you show to your child for taking his/her medications will be more important in encouraging further cooperation and responsibility for his/her treatment. If your child consistently takes his/her medications, he/she is more likely to feel better and be more active which should be rewarding for you and your child.

There are two types of privileges your child can earn: basic and special. Basic privileges include the use of the telephone, watching TV, and playing outdoors (but not off the property). Basic privileges are earned as a package, on a daily basis, and a day ahead of time. For example, if your child takes his/her medications on Monday, he/she earns basic privileges for Tuesday.

Your child can also earn special privileges depending on the number of days he/she has earned basics during the week (and you give permission). For the first week on the program, your child must earn basics on 4 of 7 days to earn a special privilege; for the second week, 5 of 7 days; for the third week, 6 of 7 days; and for the fourth week, 7 of 7 days. You and your child will come up with a list of special privileges which may include things like renting a movie, renting a video game, or going out for pizza.

To keep track of how often your child earns basics, use the attached form. This form will also help you determine if your child has earned basics on the number of days required per week to earn a special privilege. Posting this form on the refrigerator will help you and your child to remember to fill it out. Also, it will remind you to praise your child and to award privileges for taking his/her medications.

Fig. 5.4 A token-system program for improving adherence. *Source*: Michael Rapoff, PhD. University of Kansas Medical Center, Department of Pediatrics, 3901 Rainbow Blvd., Kansas City, KS. 66160–7330; 1998

What if your child does not earn basics? This means that he/she can not engage in basic privileges for the next day and is restricted to doing homework, school related reading, and regular jobs and chores that you may assign. If your child to take his/her medictions the next day in order to earn basics for the following day. However, it is vital that your child not be allowed to engage in basic privileges he/she has not earned. Children sometimes get upset about this but do not give in and let your child engage in privileges he/she has not earned. Also, avoid nagging or lecturing your child. This makes things worse.

Weekly Privilege Summary

Instructions: For each day, record the date, whether basic privileges have been earned for the next day, and your initials. At the end of the week, add up the total number of days basics were earned and whether you child met his/her weekly goal for earning a special privilege.

DAY AND DATE	BASICS EARNED? (circle one): Y= Yes; N= No	PARENT INITIALS
Monday / /	Y N	
Tuesday / /	Y N	
Wednesday / /	Y N	
Thursday / /	Y N	
Friday / /	Y N	
Saturday / /	Y N	
Sunday / /		

Total Number of Days Basics Earned This Week =

My child met his/her weekly goal? (Circle one): Yes No

Fig. 5.4 (continued)

They are then taught how to develop and implement written contracts, which specify what the patient agrees to do, what the parents will provide in the way of consequences for adherence (or sometimes nonadherence), and how to monitor and evaluate patient and parent participation. A generic handout that describes this process is shown in Fig. 5.5.

NEGOTIATING AND CONTRACTING FOR BEHAVIOR CHANGE
GUIDELINES FOR FAMILIES

This handout is for parents and children/adolescents who want to learn how to negotiate and contract for changes in behaviors that have a negative impact on the family. To negotiate means to "meet and discuss with another in order to reach an agreement." A contract is a written agreement of what has been worked out in negotiations. By adhering to the following guidelines, most families find that they can work out disagreements in a constructive way. Some families may need the assistance of a professional counselor, at least initially, to implement these guidelines.

HOW TO NEGOTIATE (THE FAMILY MEETING):

Chose a convenient time to meet as a family. After dinner is usually a good time since most families are together at this time and it does not compete with other activities. Take the phone off the hook to avoid interruptions and set a specific time limit for discussions. Most families meet at least one a week for about 30-60 minutes.

Avoid family meetings after there has been a big "blow-up." Wait until anger has subsided and then set a time for discussion. Choose some to lead the family meeting. (This is most often a parent.) The leader is responsible for making sure the family meeting is orderly and positive with everyone having a chance to be heard.

Several rules for effective negotiation should be followed during family meetings:

LEADER ENCOURAGES EVERYONE TO SPEAK

The leader should ask if anyone has anything to discuss. Start with one person and then go to the next. This will help to avoid confusion and give everyone a chance to be heard. Discuss one or two issues per family meeting. Don't try to solve all problems in one meeting. The leader should make sure everyone stays on task and does not shift to other issues or problems not under discussion for a particular meeting.

USE "I" MESSAGES

Family members should specify problem/complaints in a constructive and non-attacking way. For example, a parent is upset because one of the children has not been completing homework assignments. Instead of saying, "You have been irresponsible and lazy about doing your homework?" the parent might say, "I am concerned that because your homework assignments have not been getting done, your grades will suffer. I would like to see you be consistent in completing daily homework assignments." These "I" messages (the second example) are much more likely to lead to effective problem solving as compared to "YOU" messages which often lead to name-calling and defensiveness on the other person's part.

Fig. 5.5 Negotiating and contracting for behavior change.
Source: Michael Rapoff, Ph.D., 1988. University of Kansas Medical Center, Department of Pediatrics, 3901 Rainbow Blvd., Kansas City, KS. 66160–7330

COMMUNICATE CONSTRUCTIVELY

Children (and parents sometimes) may need to be reminded about how to state problems/ complaints in a constructive way. If a family member begins to state a complaint in an attacking or non-constructive way, the leader should politely interrupt the person and remind them to state the problem in a constructive way. Occasionally, (particularly when families first begin having meetings), a child or teenager may interrupt others and continue to speak in a negative way during discussions. This person can be asked to leave the meeting (for a short time) until they cool off. Most children and teenagers will correct this negative pattern if they receive constructive feedback and realize that decisions that affect them will be made without their input if they choose to be disruptive during family meetings.

OFFER SOLUTIONS

Once the specific problem has been identified in a constructive way, the person who identified the problem should suggest a possible solution. Others are then encouraged to offer their opinions.

PLAN FOR MONITORING AND EVALUATING SOLUTIONS

A plan to solve the problem should then be voted on. The plan should include a specific way to monitor how it is working and a time limit for determining if the plan has been effective.

DEVELOP WRITTEN CONTRACTS

To formalize solutions to problems, families may find it helpful to draw up a written contract which specifies the conditions of agreements reached during family meetings. The next section provides details of how to develop contracts.

Parents may find it necessary to overrule a decision made in a family meeting.

This should only be done under unusual circumstances and after the reasons have been thoroughly discussed with the children.

CONTRACTING FOR BEHAVIOR CHANGE

To be effective, contracts should be positive, mutually negotiated, and fair to all parties. Contracts should focus on specific behaviors (responsibilities) to be performed instead of vague references and descriptions. (For example, "Pick up dirty clothes in bedroom and put them in a hamper each night" is a better description than "Be more responsible about cleaning the bedroom.") Contracts should specify rewards/privileges which will be given after behaviors are performed. Specific ways to monitor the terms of the contract should be spelled out clearly. The time period that the contract is in effect should be specified. At the end of the contract period, there should be a review of the contract with modifications made as necessary. Contracts can also include a bonus for performance that exceeds some specified level and a penalty for failure to perform to some minimum level. (This is optional.)

Fig. 5.5 (continued)

SAMPLE CONTRACT

EFFECTIVE DATE: April 11, 2009

FAMILY CONTRACT FOR: John Jones and Mr. And Mrs. Jones

RESPONSIBILITIES	PRIVILEGES
John will complete the following regimen components each day: take pancreatic enzymes with each meal and snack; administer inhaled antibiotic and bronchodilator medications in the morning, in the afternoon, and in the evening; do chest physiotherapy 3 times; and take inhaled steroid medication twice per day.	If John completes his all regimen requirements each day, he can have phone and TV privileges in the evening. If John completes all his daily regimen requirements on 6 of 7 consecutive days, he can go out with his friends on Friday or Saturday night. If John completes all his daily regimen requirements on 7 of 7 consecutive days, he can go out with his friends on Friday and Saturday night.

MONITORING: Mr. or Mrs. Jones will directly observe whether John completes his daily regimen requirements at least during the first two weeks this contract is in effect. For each two consecutive week periods John completes all daily regimen requirements, Mr. of Mrs. Jones will observe on one less day until John is observed on 3 of 7 days. They will then observe periodically and at unannounced times.

BONUS: If John completes all regimen requirements each day without reminders by parents, he can use the family car on one of his weekend nights with his friends.

PENALTY: None

_____

John

_____

Mr. Jones

_____

Mrs. Jones

Fig. 5.5 (continued)

Discipline Strategies

In lecturing to medical students on the topic of medical adherence, I ask them if they have seen "bratty" behaviors on the pediatric inpatient ward among chronically ill children. Invariably they describe incidents where children with cancer or other chronic diseases are exhibiting negative behaviors and their parents respond ineffectively. I tell the medical students that we need to appreciate how difficult it is for parents of chronically (and maybe terminally) ill children to discipline their children who have enough negatives in their lives. Studies show that these parents, relative to parents of healthy children, are more likely to excuse their children's misbehavior and fail to set and enforce consistent limits (Ievers, Drotar, Dahms, Doershuk, & Stern, 1994; Walker, Garber, & Van Slyke, 1995). My colleagues and I try to explain to parents of ill children that setting and enforcing reasonable limits is vital to fostering self-discipline in their children. We emphasize to the parents that their children will need more self-discipline than healthy children because their children have to cope with the regular demands of life, as well as the consequences (such as adhering to complex regimens) of living with a chronic health problem. Clinicians need to provide parents with concrete recommendations for effective discipline.

So what is "effective discipline?" There is general agreement that skilled or effective discipline involves the following: (1) a positive environment that promotes appropriate behavior; (2) regular monitoring of children's behavior; (3) ignoring trivial or minor problems; (4) structuring the environment and redirecting children to more appropriate choices; (5) consistent consequences for negative behaviors (such as time-out or other sanctions); and (6) following up. In contrast, undesirable discipline involves inconsistency, noncontingent consequences, harsh punishment, and negative parental demeanor (Cipani, 2004; Socolar et al., 1997). Clinicians need to emphasize to parents that effective discipline is not just punishment for negative behaviors. However, in spite of parents' best efforts to provide positive consequences for appropriate behavior, all children (even those with chronic diseases) have to contact negative consequences for misbehavior at times (which may include refusing to adhere to their medical regimens).

For younger children, my colleagues and I often recommend using time-out (less than 10 years of age) for outright refusals to complete regimen tasks (and oppositional and aggressive behavior in general). The basic format of time-out is familiar to most readers, but our protocol for time-out, specifically for medical nonadherence, can be found in Fig. 5.6. For older children, we recommend response cost procedures, such as token fines and brief "grounding" periods, which can be reduced by completing extra chores. However, these negative consequences should only be considered when other strategies previously described (e.g., reducing negative side effects and positive incentives) have been attempted and found to be inadequate to improve adherence.

Using Time-Out for Medical Nonadherence: Guidelines for Parents

Time-out is a discipline strategy to reduce negative behaviors. It involves placing your child in a dull place for a short time immediately following an unacceptable behavior. Time-out is generally used with children from 18 months to 10 years. It is effective in reducing problem behaviors such as tantrums, hitting, not minding, and many others. Time-out works best when combined with positive attention and other consequences for appropriate behaviors.

This handout describes the use of time-out when children refuse to take medications, do special exercises, or follow other treatments that have been prescribed by a physician or therapist (so called, "medical nonadherence"). If children do not follow their medical treatments consistently, they may not get the full benefits of therapy. They may even become more seriously ill or disabled by their illness.

Please note that time-out for medical nonadherence should only be used when other techniques have been tried, such as making the regimens easier to follow, reducing negative side-effects of regimens, and educating children about their illness and treatment.

A.   Preparing to Use Time-out

1. Purchase a small portable kitchen timer.
2. Select a place for time-out–such as a chair in the kitchen. It needs to be a dull but *not* scary or dangerous place. Make sure it is a place where your child can't see the TV or play with toys.
3. There needs to be agreement between all caregivers in the home about how to use time-out and when to use it.

B.   Practicing Time-out

1. Before using time-out, discuss it with your child during a time he or she is not in trouble.
2. Tell your child there are two rules when in time-out:
   Rule 1: The time will start only when your child is quiet. If your child yells, cries, talks, or says bad words, the timer is reset as soon as he or she is quiet.
   Rule 2: If your child leaves time-out before you let him or her, you will lead him or her back to time-out without saying anything and restart the time when he or she is quiet.
3. After explaining the rules and having your child repeat them, do a practice time-out to make sure he or she understands the rules.

C. Steps for Doing Time-out

Step 1: If your child refuses to take his or her medicine (for example), say to your child, "You are not taking your medicine like I asked you to, you have to go to time-out." Say this calmly and only once. Don't threaten or warn your child. If your child does not go to time-out right away, physically guide him or her to time-out. This may mean walking with your child, taking your child by the hand and leading him or her, or (for little ones) carrying him or her to time-out.

Fig. 5.6 Time-out handout for medical nonadherence.
Source: Michael Rapoff, PhD., University of Kansas Medical Center, Department of Pediatrics, 3901 Rainbow Blvd., Kansas City, KS. 66160-7330; E-mail: mrapoff@kumc

Step 2: When your child is sitting in time-out quietly, set the time for a specific number of minutes. A good rule of thumb is a maximum of 1 minute of *quiet* for each year of life. A 2-year-old would have 2 minutes; a 3-year-old, 3 minutes; and a 5-year-old, 5 minutes.

For children over 5 years, the maximum quiet time is still 5 minutes. If your child makes noises, talks, screams, or cries, reset the time without saying a single word to your child. Do this each time he or she makes any sounds. If your child leaves time-out before the quiet time is up, lead him or her back to ime-out and restart the time.

Step 3: After your child has finished time-out, go to him or her and say, "You have been quiet, would you like to get out now?" Your child has to say yes or nod his or her head. If he or she refuses, then restart the time. Don't say this from across the room.

Step 4: After time-out is over, ask your child if he or she is ready to take the medicine (or do other things the doctor or therapist prescribed). If he or she still refuses, place him or her back in time-out and repeat steps 1, 2, and 3. If your child takes his or her medicine, praise him or her and give other rewards you may have agreed to provide.

D.   Special Problems

- *What if your child takes medicine but then spits it out or throws it up?* Check with your doctor about giving another dose (especially if your child swallows some of the medicine). In most cases, you can just give a replacement dose after time-out.
- *What if a brother or sister teases or gives attention to the child in time-out?* Make them take the child's place in time-out. That usually stops them from teasing or giving attention to the child in time-out.
- *What if your child gets so upset in time-out that it makes his or her illness worse?* Check with your child's doctor. In most cases, children should be required to finish time-out as outlined above. In rare cases, medical treatment (such as inhaler medications for children with asthma) may be necessary before resuming the time-out.

Source: Michael Rapoff, PhD., University of Kansas Medical Center, Department of Pediatrics, 3901 Rainbow Blvd., Kansas City, KS. 66160-7330; E-mail: mrapoff@kumc

Fig. 5.6 (continued)

Self-Management Strategies

A variety of strategies can be described under the rubric of self-management, including goal setting, monitoring, and self-administered consequences. Two general strategies will be highlighted here: problem solving and cognitive restructuring.

Children with chronic diseases are faced with many challenges that require effective problem-solving skills, which generally involve the following steps: (1) recognizing and defining the problem; (2) generating possible solutions; (3) developing and implementing a plan; (4) evaluating the outcome of the plan; and (5) revising or selecting another plan if unsuccessful. These skills are especially important as children move into adolescence and are faced with peer influences and social situations that may be lead them to compromise their health. Problem solving can be rehearsed with patients using standard or patient-generated vignettes. For example, the following vignette relates to glucose testing for patients with diabetes (from Thomas et al., 1997, p. 559):

"Now, imagine that your friends ask you to a video game arcade, and it's almost time for you to test your glucose. You don't have your test materials with you, and your friends are impatient to leave. If you stop and test, they will leave without you."

Patients can also be asked to keep a diary to identify situations where they are tempted to make compromises related to their regimens that can have deleterious effects on their health. They can then cycle through the problem-solving steps to come up with a plan for managing these challenges.

Cognitive (Kendall, 1993) and contemporary behavior (Hayes, 1989) theories emphasize the influence of thoughts or self-generated rules on behavior. Cognitive processes can contribute to adherence problems in two general ways: (1) patients and/or families can fail to generate rules or thoughts about diseases and regimens when it would be helpful to do so (such as "I need to take my medications consistently to give them a chance to work."); or (2) patients and/or families may generate counterproductive rules or thoughts (such as "I'll take my medicine depending on how I feel."). When patients fail to generate helpful thoughts, clinicians can assist them by suggesting helpful thoughts or rules that support better adherence to medical regimens. When they generate unhelpful thoughts, clinicians can help patients challenge or test the validity of these thoughts and substitute more helpful ways to think about their diseases and medical treatments. Clinicians need to recognize the importance of context when teaching patients and their families cognitive restructuring techniques. Table 5.3 provides examples of adherence-relevant thoughts and the contexts under which these thoughts can lead to positive or negative outcomes for patients.

Psychotherapeutic Interventions

In some cases, medical nonadherence can be embedded in, or exist concurrently with, more serious patient or family problems (Rapoff & Barnard, 1991). For some patients, this may be part of a broader pattern of externalizing (e.g., oppositional behavior) or internalizing (e.g., depression) problems. There may also be significant parental or family problems (e.g., parental depression, marital conflict, or abuse). Children with chronic health problems and their parents are at risk for psychologic morbidity and most do not receive necessary mental health services (Bauman,

Table 5.3 Adherence-related thoughts about treatments and diseases that can have positive or negative consequences

Thought	Possible positive consequences	Possible negative consequences
"I take my medicine depending on how I feel; sometimes more, sometimes less"	Useful guide for PRN (as needed) medications, if the person can appropriately match with symptoms	Failure to achieve therapeutic drug level for continuous regimens
"This medicine is causing harm or making me feel worse"	Could avoid potentially serious side effects	Premature discontinuation of effective treatment (especially when side effects are not serious, temporary, and can be minimized)
"This medicine (treatment) is not helping"	Discuss with provider and treatment is modified or other treatments are added	Premature discontinuation of effective treatment, (especially if insufficient time has elapsed to judge efficacy)
"I don't really have this disease."	If true, then avoids unnecessary treatments with possible negative side effects	If false, heightens the potential for decreased quantity and quality of life
"My disease is not that bad"	If true, then unnecessary treatments are avoided	If false, heightens the potential for decreased quantity and quality of life

Drotar, Leventhal, Perrin, & Pless, 1997). Psychosocial problems may need to be addressed before or concurrent with efforts to manage medical nonadherence by mental health professionals who have extensive experience with children and families in medical settings. However, underlying patient or family dysfunction is rarely the primary contributor to medical nonadherence and providers would do well to look elsewhere unless their evaluation reveals the presence of significant patient or family dysfunction.

In rare cases, nonadherence to medications by parents for life-threatening diseases affecting their young children has been considered medical neglect. A study conducted at Arkansas Children's Hospital identified six patients with HIV who had high viral loads despite having documented sensitivity to antiretroviral medications and their caregivers reported that they were giving medications regularly (Roberts et al., 2004). These six families were exposed to a three-step intervention: (1) a home health-care nurse made home visits to provide support at least 2 times per week for at least 2 weeks; (2) the child was hospitalized for 4 days to directly administer medications and further educate and support caregivers; and (3) failing the other two steps, a physician-initiated medical neglect report was made to the Arkansas Department of Human Services. Caregivers of four of the six children responded to the intervention after step 2 and the remaining two were placed in foster care with subsequent improvements in viral load. These are considered to be extreme cases, but do set a precedent for considering life-threatening nonadherence by caretakers of young children as medical neglect.

Summary of Behavioral Strategies

There are a number of cognitive-behavior change strategies available to assist patients and their families to improve and sustain adherence to medical regimens. They have been found to be the most effective adherence-improvement strategies, particularly for chronic disease regimens (Rapoff & Barnard, 1991). However, clinicians must be careful to individualize interventions to address the unique environmental and cognitive contexts of specific patients and their families.

Individualizing Interventions: Barriers to Adherence and Functional Analysis

Whether a particular strategy or set of strategies is effective in a given clinical context depends on how well variables relevant for an individual patient and family have been identified and can be modified to improve adherence. Indeed, "one size does not fit all." Clinicians need to individualize interventions to address the unique environmental and person-related factors that impact adherence. Two such strategies will be discussed here: (1) addressing unique "barriers" or obstacles to adherence and (2) functional analysis or identifying functional relationships that are applicable to particular behaviors for particular patients and their families.

Barriers to Adherence

The purpose of this approach is to obtain patient and family perspectives on potential events or situations, which may interfere with adequate adherence. This can be done by structured interviews, questionnaires, or having patients keep written diaries. An example of a standard set of barriers from the Barriers to Adherence Interview for children (over 10 years old) with asthma or cystic fibrosis and their parents is presented in Fig. 5.7 (Modi & Quittner, 2006a). Parents and children are first asked to identify barriers to regimen components (e.g., airway clearance, nebulized medications, inhaler use, etc., for cystic fibrosis) and to rate how often a barrier occurs and how difficult it is, on a 5-point scale, with 1 = "not at all" and 5 = "a lot." They are then presented the list of 25 barriers in Fig. 5.7 and asked to identify any additional barriers from the list and rate frequency and difficulty for each barrier endorsed. Barriers were quite similar by illness and informant, with the most common barriers being forgetting, oppositional behaviors, and difficulties with time management. Although not statistically significant, moderate negative correlations were found between the barriers measure and parent and child self-report, pharmacy refill, phone diary, and electronic monitoring measures of adherence (Modi & Quittner, 2006a).

If standard barrier measures are not available for a particular illness, clinicians can conduct clinical interviews with patients and their families. For example, my colleagues and I routinely interview patients and their parents separately and ask "What gets in the way of you taking your medicines (or doing exercises, following

BARRIERS ADHERENCE INTERVIEW ANSWER CHOICES

_____1. Forgetting (to take medications or bring them with you/picking up from pharmacy) _____2. Dislike tastes _____3. Other Side effects (e.g. bad taste, heart racing, nausea) _____4. Hard to swallow _____5. Not sure the medication works or is needed _____6. Difficult to understand doctor's instructions/Doctor's advice _____7. Expensive _____8. Embarrassing/Don't want to take them in front of friends _____9. Too many medications _____10. Too busy or takes too much time/can't find the time/scheduling problems _____12. Started feeling better _____13. Lost medication _____14. Wants to be normal _____15. Ran out of medications/Pharmacy ran out _____16. Family emergencies _____17. Oppositional behaviors (refuses, not wanting to do it, tired of meds, won't take them, play/watch tv) _____18. Difficult to incorporate needs into family life/Other caregivers supervising _____19. Can't take medications/device with you when you are out _____21. Tired/Don't feel well _____22. Technique problems _____23. Machine is too bulky/loud or uncomfortable mask/device _____24. Doesn't need the medication _____25. Eating/Feeding issues (e.g. feels full, rushes eating)

Fig. 5.7 Identifying barriers to adherence to asthma and cystic fibrosis regimens. Reprinted from Modi and Quittner (2006a) with permission by Oxford University Press

your diet, etc.)?" One young man with JRA I interviewed mentioned several barriers related to taking his anti-inflammatory medication: (1) it was harder to remember to take his medications when he was not hurting; (2) when he was under time pressures in the morning to get ready for school and catch the school bus, he sometimes forget; (3) when he got back home late in the evening from after-school activities, he was tired, ate supper, and after he went to bed, he did not want to get out of bed even if he remembered he had not taken his evening dose; and (4) he admitted that when he was angry with his parents, he would not take his medicine to "get back at my parents."

Once information has been obtained about barriers to adherence unique to a particular patient and family, interventions can be designed to overcome these specific barriers. For example, clinicians can engage patients in problem solving to identify potential ways to reduce barriers. With the above-mentioned patient with JRA, we strategized about several options to overcome barriers, such as prompting himself to take medications by setting his watch alarm and ways to manage his anger toward his parents without compromising his health (e.g., conflict resolution and cognitive restructuring of anger-inducing thoughts).

Functional Analysis

This strategy involves identifying relevant, modifiable, and (potentially) causal variables that are applicable to a specified set of target behaviors for particular patients and their families (Friman, 2009; Haynes & O'Brien, 1990). Although this approach has been historically aligned with applied behavior analysis (see special issue, *Journal of Applied Behavior Analysis*, 1994, volume 27, number 2), its applicability has been extended to clinical psychology in general (Sturmey, 1996; Yoman, 2008). The following steps for conducting a functional analysis can be gleaned from the literature:

- Target behaviors are operationally defined.
- Antecedent events that predict the occurrence or nonoccurrence of target behaviors are identified. Hypotheses are developed concerning the consequences that maintain behaviors (or could maintain behaviors, in the case of low-rate appropriate behaviors), which are of two major types: to obtain something desirable or to avoid/escape something undesirable.
- Direct observational data are collected when possible to provide at least correlational confirmation of hypotheses about antecedent and consequent events (Horner, 1994; O'Neill, Horner, Albin, Storey, & Sprague, 1990).

Contrary to misconceptions about applied behavior analysis, private events (such as thoughts, feelings, and physiological events) can be entered into a functional analysis as target behaviors (e.g., pain intensity), antecedent events (e.g., dysfunctional thoughts), or consequent events (e.g., pain reduction as consequence of taking medications). However, private events are not afforded any special status compared to other variables.

Information for a functional analysis can be obtained by structured interviews, questionnaires, or (preferably) by direct observation over extended periods of time (see O'Neill et al., 1990 for examples of each). Results of the functional analysis are then clinically or experimentally tested by modifying antecedent and consequent conditions and assessing the effects on target behaviors (Allen & Warzak, 2000). For example, my colleagues and I worked with a 7-year-old girl with severe JRA, who was nonadherent to medications, wearing wrist or knee splints at night, and doing a prone lying exercise to prevent hip contractures (Rapoff et al., 1984). Extensive interviews with this patient and her parents and direct observations in the home were conducted to identify relevant variables which contributed to her nonadherence. Antecedent conditions identified included proximal or more specific events (e.g., mother having to excessively prompt and "nag" the child to adhere) and more molar events (e.g., large family with limited financial resources and a mother who felt "overwhelmed" with general child-rearing tasks and stressors of having to care for a child with a severely limiting disease). Consequent conditions identified included the lack of positive consequences for adherence (e.g., child was ignored when she was adherent because she was doing "what was expected" of her) and the almost exclusive reliance on verbal reprimands as a consequence for nonadherence. A token reinforcement and time-out program was implemented to address these antecedent and consequent conditions, and we assisted the family in finding financial support for medical and psychosocial services. Also, we worked with the mother on establishing effective child-rearing skills with all her children. This intervention was effective in improving adherence to each regimen component and there was some evidence for improvement in joint function.

Technology-Based Interventions

Children, adolescents, and their parents are very savvy when it comes to understanding and using technology, such as computer games, hand-held devices (PDAs, cell phones), and the World Wide Web. A survey by the Pew Foundation, in August 2006, found that 70% of American households had Internet access (Pew Internet & American Life Project, 2006). Adolescents in particularly around the world are comfortable using the Internet as a source of health information (Borzekowski, Fobil, & Kofi, 2006; Gray, Klein, Noyce, Sesselberg, & Cantrill, 2005). In designing interventions to improve adherence, we need to take advantage of emerging technologies to reach more patients and their families and to engage them in finding ways to enhance adherence and health outcomes.

CD-ROM or Web-based interventions offer several advantages: (1) they can be highly structured, thus enhancing treatment fidelity; (2) they can also be tailored to the specific barriers patients and families are facing; (3) more patients and families can have access to adherence interventions from their homes; (4) engaging elements such as audio, animation, and interactivity can be built into these programs to make them more attractive and encourage adherence to the adherence interventions; (5) with Web-based programs, outcome assessments can be online and use of the programs can be monitored in real time (Drotar et al., 2006; Ritterband et al., 2003).

There are, however, a number of barriers that need to be addressed when using technology-based interventions: (1) we need to make sure patients and families are proficient in using programs; (2) confidentiality is a significant issue and information conveyed over the Web must be protected; (3) technology-based interventions are expensive to develop and require a multidisciplinary team consisting of pediatric psychologists, physicians, nurses, other allied health-care professionals, computer and Web programmers, graphic artists, health informatics evaluators, and statisticians for database development; (4) the use of technology must be monitored for quality control purposes; and (5) the programs need to be easy to use and avoid putting excess burdens on patients, their families, or health-care provider (Drotar et al., 2006; Fisher & Fried, 2003; Ritterband et al., 2003).

CD-ROM and Web-based programs and games have been developed for patients with asthma, cystic fibrosis, and type 1 diabetes (Brown et al., 1997; Davis, Quittner, Stack, & Yang, 2004; Krishna et al., 2003; McPherson, Glazebrook, Forster, James, & Smyth, 2006; Rubin et al., 1986). In general, these programs produce significant increases in knowledge of diseases and treatments, but no significant effects on health outcomes. The studies on these programs do not measure adherence directly. This should not be surprising given the content of these programs. For example, the Starlight Foundation asthma program, "Quest for the Code," is designed for children and teens 7–15 years and covers the following topics: early warning signs and symptoms, identifying and avoiding triggers, myths about asthma, how asthma affects the lungs, proper use of asthma-medication devices, long-term control medicine and quick-relief medicine, measuring and monitoring peak flow, and how to answer questions from peers about asthma. The program is very engaging and includes voice-overs by famous actors. What are missing from this and other programs are specific strategies for enhancing adherence. For example, patients and families can select from a list of barriers and the program would have branching capabilities to guide them to specific strategies for overcoming the barriers they endorsed. In Table 5.4, I present the essential elements of a CD-ROM or Web-based program for enhancing adherence resulting from a brainstorming dialogue.

Another potentially useful technology for enhancing adherence is telehealth, which has been used with patients with asthma and type 1 diabetes (Chan et al., 2007; Heidgerken et al., 2006; Gelfand, Geffken, Halsey-Lyda, Muir, & Malasanos, 2003). Although telehealth interventions have not been studied extensively, one program for children with asthma was a randomized control trial and showed significantly better inhaler technique and significantly higher adherence compared

Table 5.4 Essential elements of a CD-ROM or Web-based program for enhancing adherence to pediatric medical regimens

1. It would be individualized by type of disease and developmental level of patients.
2. It would include an educational component:
    a. Type of disease
    b. How doctors diagnose
    c. Causes/triggers
    d. Course of disease/prognosis (being careful about discussing long-term complications)
    e. Recommended treatments and what they are intended to accomplish
    f. Potential negative side effects and how they can be minimized
    g. Importance of consistent adherence
    h. Chalkboards online where children and parents can talk with each other
3. It would include a behavioral component:
    a. Having patient/family discuss with provider how to simplify regimen and reducing side effects if they appear
    b. Cueing/prompting (calendars, text messages, watch alarms) and assessing if strategies were used
    c. Monitoring adherence to regimen components (self and parents)
    d. Having incentives for adherence (point system, contracts) and confirming they have adhered to the program
    e. Addressing barriers to adherence and problem solving
    f. Having disincentives for nonadherence (time-out for younger children, loss of points, brief loss of privileges)
    g. Addressing regimen-related thoughts that may be helpful or not in promoting adherence (e.g., "I feel ok, so I don't need to take my medicine")
    h. If electronic monitoring is available, downloading periodically and giving feedback to patients and families (e.g., bar graph showing % adherence for past two weeks)

Table 5.4 (continued)

---

    i. Monitoring symptoms and linking these to adherence
    j. Having booster sessions online and determining the timing of these
    k. Allowing families to have the ability to access strategies even after completing the program
    l. Including family- and patient-only sessions within the program
    m. Including communication and problem-solving training
    n. Addressing how responsibility is allocated within the family for implementing regimen components
    o. Monitoring changes in treatment plans for individual patients to make sure they are up to date and agree with their provider's recommendations

4. It would need to be flashy, attractive to patients, have good graphics and music, not too wordy, and embed opportunities for patients to respond (answer questions, practice a skill like using a monitoring strategy).
    a. Would need creative people to write scripts and choose graphics and music
    b. Would need information technology people to program
    c. Mix up of child and adult voiceovers for recording of the script
    d. Expert review of content and focus groups with families in developing the programs

---

Source: With appreciation to Drs. Lori Stark, Denny Drotar, Korey Hood, Kevin Hommell, Avani Modi, and Ahna Pai at Cincinnati Children's Hospital Medical Center for graciously hosting me as a Visiting Professor during my sabbatical leave in 2008 and helping me come up with this list.

to office-based care (Chan et al., 2007). Patients and families could be provided Webcams to communicate with providers and strategize about how to enhance adherence and disease self-management.

Conclusions

Interventions for improving adherence to medical regimens are often suggested in the literature, but there is clearly a need to individualize these interventions based on an assessment of the unique personal, family, social, and environmental factors that are present for particular patients and families. Such a thorough assessment will better equip clinicians to identify educational approaches, changes in health-care delivery, and behavior change strategies, which may be helpful in improving adherence. We also need to take advantage of existing technologies, like the Web, and include educational information and specific strategies for enhancing adherence and health outcomes. There is much to be done in this area as few intervention studies have been reported in the literature. The adherence-intervention literature will now be reviewed and recommendations for future research and clinical directions will be offered.

Chapter 6
Review of Adherence Intervention Studies and Top Ten Ways to Advance Research on Adherence to Pediatric Medical Regimens

Since the first edition of this book, there are encouraging signs that researchers are not limiting themselves to just documenting the prevalence, correlates, and consequences of medical nonadherence. They are conducting controlled studies using randomized controlled group designs and single-subject designs to evaluate the impact of interventions on adherence and health outcomes. The purpose of this final chapter is to review and critique studies on improving adherence to regimens for acute and chronic pediatric diseases, summarize recent meta-analyses of this literature, and offer 10 ways that research on pediatric medical adherence can be improved.

Intervention Studies on Improving Adherence to Regimens for Acute Pediatric Diseases

Surprisingly, there are still not many studies that have experimentally investigated strategies for improving adherence to regimens for acute diseases, such as antibiotics in the treatment of otitis media. A total of 11 were located for this review, of which, 4 were new since the previous edition of this book (see Table 6.1). The vast majority (9 of 11; 82%) of the studies focused on adherence to antibiotic regimens for otitis media. The average sample size of these studies is 210, with a range of 33–771. Combination adherence measures (e.g., pill count plus assay) were used in six of the studies (55%), followed by pill counts in three studies (27%), and assays in two studies (18%). In terms of designs, eight of the studies (73%) were randomized controlled trials and the remainder of the studies was nonrandomized trials. Most of the interventions involved extended education and counseling about medications from a physician or pharmacy personnel and phone reminders as strategies for enhancing adherence to medications. One study also found that having parents verbally commit to dispense prescribed medications was effective in raising adherence to antibiotics for otitis media (Kulik & Carlino, 1987). Another study was also instructive in showing that continuing education programs for pediatricians that focus on strategies for improving adherence (such as simplifying regimens) can be effective in improving adherence to antibiotics for otitis media (Maiman, Becker, Liptak, Nazarian, &

M.A. Rapoff, *Adherence to Pediatric Medical Regimens*, Issues in Clinical Child
Psychology, DOI 10.1007/978-1-4419-0570-3_6,
© Springer Science+Business Media, LLC 2010

Table 6.1 Adherence intervention studies targeting acute disease regimens in pediatrics

References	Sample and disease	Regimen and Measure	Procedures	Outcome
Bertakis, 1986	$N = 59$ Otitis media	Antibiotics Medication measurement	Parents randomly assigned to intervention group (education about treatment of otitis media and its benefits) or control group (education about use of car seats)	No significant differences in adherence; 91.8% in the intervention group and 85.6% in the control group
Casey, Rosen, Glowasky, and Ludgwig, 1985	$N = 312$ 3 mos–11 yrs ($M = 2.5$ yrs) Otitis media	Antibiotic Parent report and medication measurement	Sequentially assigned to one of three intervention groups (Gr. 1 nurse education and phone call on days 2 and 13; Gr. 2 received phone calls only; Gr. 3 received nurse education session only) or two control groups (Gr. 4 completed a compliance questionnaire; Gr. 5 received no intervention and did not complete the questionnaire)	No significant differences between groups Adherence ranged from 82% for Gr. 4 to 100% for Gr. 3
Colcher and Bass, 1972	$N = 300$ (1–15 yrs) Pharyngitis	Penicillin Urine assay	Random assignment to 3 groups: Gr. 1 = penicillin injection; Gr. 2 = oral penicillin and routine instructions; Gr. 3 = oral penicillin and extended counseling regarding medication use and written instructions	Adherence by group: Gr. 1 = 87%; Gr. 2 = 58%; and Gr. 3 = 80% (significant difference between Grs 1 and 3 vs. Gr. 2). No significant difference in treatment failures. Significantly higher relapse rate in Gr. 2 vs. Grs 1 and 3.

Table 6.1 (continued)

References	Sample and disease	Regimen and Measure	Procedures	Outcome
Ellison and Altemeier, 1982	$N = 72$ $M = 12.3$ mos Otitis media	Amoxicillin Urine assay	Random assignment to use teaspoon or syringe to dispense medications	No significant difference in adherence by delivery method: teaspoon $=56\%$ and syringe $= 67\%$
Fink, Malloy, Cohen, Greycloud, and Martin, 1969	$N = 274$ Various acute illnesses	Medications Interviews and medical records	Random assignment to experimental group (special counseling by family health management specialist) or control group (usual care)	Significant difference in adherence: 69% in experimental group vs. 18% in control group
Finney, Friman, Rapoff, and Christophersen, 1985	$N = 73$ (1–12 yrs) Otitis media	Antibiotics Pill count and urine assay	Random assignment to experimental group (educational handout, monitoring, and midregimen phone reminder) or control group (standard care)	Adherence was significantly higher in experimental group (82%) vs. the control group (49%). No significant difference in resolution of otitis media.
Kulik and Carlino, 1987	$N = 89$ (1–14 yrs) Otitis media	Antibiotics Parental report (urine assay for 10 patients)	Random assignment to commitment (physician asked parents for verbal commitment to give all medications) and choice (parents could choose between two different antibiotics) manipulations	High-commitment patients had significantly higher adherence (97%) vs. low-commitment patients (91%). Choice condition not significant. No significant differences in resolution of otitis media.
Maiman et al., 1988	$N = 771$ ($M = 46$ months) Otitis media	Antibiotics Pill counts and parental report	Pediatricians randomly assigned to control or one of two continuing medical education programs: tutorial with printed materials (TPM) or mailed printed materials only (MPM). Content of education included communication of information, simplifying regimens, and modifying health beliefs.	Patients of pediatricians in TPM group significantly less likely to miss doses as assessed by pill counts; but MPM group missed significantly fewer doses as assessed by parental report

Table 6.1 (continued)

References	Sample and disease	Regimen and Measure	Procedures	Outcome
Mattar et al., 1975	$N = 233$ (1–12 yrs) Otitis media	Antibiotics Pill count	Education group ($N = 33$) compared to controls ($N = 200$); no random assignment. Education group parents given written instructions and monitoring form by pharmacy personnel	Significantly higher adherence in the education group (51%) vs. controls (8.5%)
Schwartz-Lookinland, McKeever, and Saputo, 1989	$N = 33$ (Hispanic, mother–child pairs) $M = 2.5$ yrs Otitis media	Amoxicillin Medication measurement	Subject randomly selected, then assigned to experimental group (received written instruction handout in Spanish and a pictorial handout on correct dosing, storage of medications, etc.) or control group (verbal instructions only)	No significant differences between groups; 67.6% adherent in the experimental group and 64.5% in the control group
Williams et al., 1986	$N = 90$ (2–24 mos; $M = 7.6$ mos) Otitis media	Antibiotics Parental report, bottle measurement, and urine assay	Patients randomly assigned to one of three groups: control, slide-tape (parents shown in clinic, emphasizing importance of adherence), or follow-up phone call (parents phoned on 4th day of therapy to encourage continued adherence)	No significant differences on any adherence measure between groups

Rounds, 1988). Overall, however, only 6 of the 11 studies (55%) showed positive results on adherence and most (if they measured outcomes) failed to show a positive effect on treatment outcomes, such as resolution of otitis media.

Intervention Studies on Improving Adherence to Regimens for Chronic Pediatric Diseases

Compared to regimens for acute diseases, there are many more experimental studies, which examined the efficacy of strategies for improving adherence to chronic disease regimens. A total of 64 studies were located for this review, of which, 37 (58%) were new since the first edition of this book (see Table 6.2). Over half of these studies focused on adherence to regimens for diabetes (20/64 studies; 31%) or asthma (16/64 studies; 25%). Also, nearly half of the studies focused on adherence to medications (31/64; 48%), which is understandable given the primacy of medications in the treatment of chronic diseases. Combination adherence measures (e.g., electronic monitoring plus patient and parent report) were used in 14 of the 64 studies (22%), followed by parent report (13/64; 20%) and electronic monitoring (8/64; 13%). Encouragingly, about one-third of studies (21/64; 33%) used an assay, electronic monitoring, or direct observations, which are considered more objective measure of adherence. In terms of designs, 32 of the 64 studies (50%) were randomized controlled trials, 14 of the 64 (22%) used single-subject designs, and the remainder were nonrandomized trials.

Multicomponent education, behavioral and cognitive strategies continue to be the primary interventions tested. Educational strategies are rarely attempted in isolation, but usually combined with behavioral strategies, such as monitoring and positive reinforcement. Educational strategies alone may just have limited impact on improving adherence. Or possibly, patients selected for adherence interventions may have been exposed to educational efforts that previously failed to enhance adherence. The primary organizational strategy employed to improve adherence has been simplifying regimens. Reducing the number of daily medications did enhance adherence to medications for asthma (Tinkelman, Vanderpool, Carroll, Page, & Spangler, 1980) and JRA (Rapoff et al., 1988a).

By far the most frequently tested and effective strategies have been behaviorally based, including increased monitoring (e.g., Eney & Goldstein, 1976), explicit training and feedback (e.g., Epstein et al., 1981), contracting (e.g., Gross, 1983), and reward systems (e.g., Stark et al., 2005a,b). There have also been advancements in developing and testing behavioral family systems-based interventions that focus on the entire family and involve communication training, problem-solving, cognitive restructuring, and behavioral contracting (e.g., Wysocki & Gavin, 2006).

One of the more intriguing studies reviewed in Table 6.2 employed a parent simulation component (Satin, La Greca, Zigo, & Skyler, 1989). Parents of children with insulin-dependent diabetes simulated their children's regimen by (1) injecting themselves twice daily with normal saline; (2) testing and recording urinary glucose and ketones; (3) following a meal plan, including avoiding concentrated sweets; (4) following an exercise plan; (5) recording "hypoglycemic" episodes (missing or delaying meals and snacks or failing to consume extra snacks with extra activity); and (6) submitting to a blood test for glycosylated hemoglobin. After the simulation period, the parents were asked about difficulties they encountered in following the simulated regimen and how this affected the way they viewed their teenager with diabetes. Simulation coupled with weekly support and educational sessions resulted in improvements in metabolic control relative to a control group. Simulations have also been added to behavioral family systems-based interventions (e.g., Wysocki & Gavin, 2006) and they have been employed with medical students (Kastrissios et al., 1996) and physicians and nurses (Morse, Simon, & Balson, 1993) to increase their awareness of barriers to adherence and address these barriers with their patients.

Of the 64 studies in Table 6.2, 45 (70%) reported positive effects on enhancing adherence (either statistically significant between-group differences or convincing graphic displays of single-subject data). Another 10 studies (16%) showed no significant or obvious effect on adherence and the remaining 9 studies (14%) showed mixed results (interventions were not immediately beneficial or the gains were not maintained after the intervention was delivered).

Meta-Analytic Reviews of Adherence Interventions for Pediatric Medical Regimens

Qualitative reviews, as in the previous section of this chapter, cannot determine the quantitative power and effectiveness of adherence interventions. A meta-analysis is the best technique to provide such information (Rosenthal, 1991). Because adherence is a continuous variable, the recommended effect size (ES) estimate is the standardized mean difference effect size, also known as the d statistic (Lipsey & Wilson, 2001). The d statistic is the difference between the means (M1–M2) divided by the pooled standard deviation. If M1 is the experimental group mean and M2 is the control group mean, then the difference is positive if it is in the direction of greater adherence in the experimental group. If d is equal to zero, then the distribution of scores for the experimental group overlaps completely with the distribution of scores for the control group. Cohen (1988) classified d statistics as follows:

- "Small," $d = 0.20$ (14.7% nonoverlap)
- "Medium," $d = 0.50$ (33% nonoverlap)
- "Large," $d = 0.80$ (47.4% nonoverlap)

Meta-Analyses of Adherence Interventions for Adults

Several reviews and meta-analytic reviews have been published on adherence interventions for adults (Haynes, McKibbon, & Kanani, 1996; Haynes, Ackloo, Sahota,

Table 6.2 Adherence intervention studies for chronic pediatric diseases

References	Sample	Regimen/measure	Procedures	Outcome
		Asthma		
Baum and Creer (1986)	$N = 16$ 6–16 yrs	Theophylline Pill counts by parents	Random assignment to self-monitoring group or self-monitoring + education	No significant between-group differences on adherence
Bonner et al. (2002)	$N = 119$ 4.2–19.1 yrs ($M = 9.5$ yrs) Specifically recruited Latino and African-American families	Medications Caregivers interviewed (4 items assessing "family adherence," such as administering medications as prescribed; 0 to 4 range with higher scores = higher adherence)	Random assignment to control (usual care) or intervention (three group workshops at 1-month intervals and phone calls between workshops; training to use asthma diaries and peak flow meters, importance of controller medications based on asthma symptoms, and following action plans for managing asthma)	Family adherence significantly higher at follow-up for the intervention vs. control group (M's = 3.14 vs. 2.14; $p < 0.001$; effect size = 0.79)
Burkhart, Dunbar-Jacob, Fireman, and Rohay (2002)	$N = 42$ 7–11 yrs ($M = 9.6$ yrs)	Peak Expiratory Flow Rate (PEFR) monitoring Electronic monitor	Random assignment to usual care or intervention (contingency management including contracts, reinforcement, tailoring, and reminders)	PEFR monitoring at the end of the 5-wk trial was higher (but not significantly) for the intervention vs. control group (M's = 70.6%, 62.9%, respectively)
Burkhart, Rayens, Oakley, Abshire, and Zhang, (2007)	$N = 77$ 7–12 yrs ($M = 9$ yrs)	Peak Expiratory Flow Rate (PEFR) monitoring Electronic monitor	Random assignment to intervention (5 sessions on peak flow use, contingency management, including contracts, self-monitoring, reinforcing, tailoring, and cueing) or control group (3 sessions with education on peak flow monitoring and other	No significant differences at week 8 (postintervention); intervention group Mdn = 86% and control group Mdn = 71% Intervention group higher at week 16 (Mdn =71%) vs. control group (Mdn =57%; $p = 0.05$)

Table 6.2 (continued)

References	Sample	Regimen/measure	Procedures	Outcome
Chan et al. (2007)	$N = 120$ 6–17 yrs	Inhaled steroids Pharmacy refill Symptom diaries (completed by patients)	education, but no contingency management components) Random assignment to office-based (traditional in-person education and case management) or virtual group (received computers, Internet connections, in-home Internet-based education and case management via study Web site) over a 12-mo period	No differences between groups on adherence to inhaled steroids Significantly greater diaries completed in the virtual group (35.4%) vs. the office-based group (20.8%) No differences between groups in ER visits, hospitalizations, unscheduled asthma-related clinic visits, pulmonary function, asthma knowledge scores, or quality of life
da Costa et al. (1997)	$N = 2$ 8 and 10 yrs	Inhaled corticosteroids Electronic monitor	Withdrawal design Following baseline, patients given education and token system intervention, followed by withdrawal of intervention	Education and token system improved adherence and withdrawal, and reinstatement of token system for one patient demonstrated effectiveness of the token system Some improvements in pulmonary function for one patient
Eney and Goldstein (1976)	$N = 90$ 3–16 yrs	Theophylline Serum/salivary assays	Random selection, but not assignment to 2 groups: Group 1 had no specific intervention. Group 2 patients informed that drug ingestion was being monitored and physicians were more "directive" in discussing adherence	11% of patients in Group 1 had therapeutic drug levels vs. 42% in Group 2

Table 6.2 (continued)

References	Sample	Regimen/measure	Procedures	Outcome
Kamps et al. (2008)	$N = 15$ 7–12 years	Inhaled steroids Electronic monitor	Random assignment to treatment or comparison group. Both groups received 6 weekly sessions (~60 min in length per session) in the home. The treatment group received weekly feedback on downloaded adherence data from the monitor plus education, self-monitoring, a point system, barriers identification, and problem-solving and cognitive restructuring strategies. The comparison group received education plus communication and relaxation training and coping strategies for stress.	Pooled time series analysis indicated that the treatment group significantly increased their adherence during the intervention phase (by 16.38%) while the comparison group did not. However, these gains for the treatment group were not maintained after the intervention phase. There were no significant between-group differences on secondary measures of quality of life, pulmonary function, or total health-care costs.
LeBaron, Zeltzer, Ratner, and Kniker (1985)	$N = 31$ 6–17 yrs ($M = 10.6$ yrs)	Cromolyn sodium Self-report (0–10 scale, with 0= "totally noncompliant, not taken at all" and 10= "totally compliant, taken all times as prescribed") Urine assay at each monthly visit	Random assignment to education group (nurse gave instructions on proper use of medication and had patients demonstrate use, over 3 visits) or usual care	No significant differences between groups on self-reported adherence. Mean ratings for the education group increased significantly from 6.21 at visit 2 to 8.64 at visit 5 ($p < 0.025$). No significant differences between groups on positive urine assays. Patient report and results of urine assay agreed 85% of the time.

Table 6.2 (continued)

References	Sample	Regimen/measure	Procedures	Outcome
Lewis, Rachelefsky, Lewis, de la Sota, and Kaplan (1984)	$N = 76$ 7–12 yrs ($M = 10$ yrs)	Medications Parent report ("Who remembers to take extra medicine when necessary?")	Random assignment to control group (three 90-min group sessions covering asthma, medications, and relaxation exercises) or Asthma Care Training (ACT; five 60-min sessions covering asthma, medications, relaxation exercises, and emphasizing increased self-care role for children)	No differences at 1-year posttest on knowledge and perceived severity of asthma Proportion of parents reporting that their child remembered to take extra medicine when necessary significantly increased in the ACT group (40–56%, $p < 0.05$) vs. the control group (26.3–37.5%, NS)
Marosi and Stiesmeyer (2001)	$N = 80$ ($M = 12.9$ yrs)	Inhaled medications Self-report	One group, pre-posttest design. Intervention included written asthma management plan, enhanced education, and phone contact with nurse to resolve adherence difficulties.	At initial visit, adherence was 40% and increased to 75% at 6-mo follow-up
Rubin et al. (1986)	$N = 54$ 7–12 yrs ($M = 9$ yrs)	Parent and child report (Asthma Behavioral Assessment Questionnaire, assessing behaviors related to management of asthma)	Random assignment to experimental group ("Asthma Command" computer game, covering recognition of symptoms, appropriate use of medications, appropriate use of ER and clinic visits, and encouragement of school attendance) or control group (nonasthma-related computer	Participants in the experimental group scored significantly higher on the child Asthma Behavioral Assessment questionnaire ($p < 0.008$). No differences between groups on acute visits due to asthma, hospital days, or school absences.

Table 6.2 (continued)

References	Sample	Regimen/measure	Procedures	Outcome
Smith, Seale, Ley, Shaw, and Braes (1986)	$N = 196$ 5–16 yrs	Medications Parent and physician ratings	game); all participants attended 45-min sessions every 6 wks for 10 mos Pretest, posttest control group design. Intervention group received educational and behavioral strategies (written information, tailoring of regimen, and increased monitoring).	Significantly higher adherence for the intervention group (78%) vs. the control group (55%)
Smith, Seale, Ley, Mellis, and Shaw (1994)	$N = 53$ 5–15 yrs	Medications Investigator ratings	One group, pre-post test design. Baseline followed by educational and behavioral strategies (written information, tailoring of regimen, and increased monitoring)	Significant increase in adherence from pre- (73%) to post- (83%) assessment. Significant improvement in asthma severity and pulmonary function
Tinkelman et al., (1980)	$N = 20$ 11–18 yrs	Theophylline Serum assay and pill counts	Random assignment to short-acting (q 6 hr) or sustained-release (q 12 hrs) theophylline. Dosing instructions given for both preparations.	Significantly higher adherence with sustained-release vs. short-acting theophylline by pill counts. No significant difference in serum levels
van Es , Nagelkerke, Colland, Scholten, and Bouter, (2001)	$N = 112$ 11–18 yrs $(M = 14$ yrs)	Inhaled steroid Patient report (10-point scale, where $1 = $ "never take medications" to $10 = $ "always take medications")	Random assignment to control (usual care) or intervention group. Intervention involved 4 individual sessions with a nurse and 3 group sessions over a 1-year period. Topics covered	No significant differences on adherence between groups at immediate follow-up (7.8 for intervention group and 7.3 for the control group; $p = 0.14$) and trend for higher adherence in the

Table 6.2   (continued)

References	Sample	Regimen/measure	Procedures	Outcome
			included the proper technique for inhaled medication, information on medications, talking with doctor and peers about asthma, attitude toward asthma and medications, and refusing to accept a cigarette.	intervention group (7.7) vs. the control group (6.7) at 24-mo follow-up ($p = 0.05$)
			Cardiac	
Gordis and Markowitz (1971)	$N = 17$	Prophylactic penicillin Urine assay	Random assignment to two groups: continuous care (same physician, increased accessibility, and comprehensive care) and specialty care (different physicians seen and treated only for rheumatic fever)	No significant differences between groups on adherence
			Cystic fibrosis	
Bartholomew et al. (1997)	$N = 199$ <1–18 yrs ($M = 8.6$ yrs)	Regimen not specified Self-Management Questionnaire for Cystic Fibrosis (caregiver and adolescent versions)	Nonequivalent comparison (usual care) group design vs. intervention (CF Family Education Program), including education and goal setting, reinforcement, modeling, skill training, and self-monitoring	Significantly higher improvement in self-management in the intervention group vs. usual care for both caregiver and adolescent reports (p's < 0.05; effect sizes 0.36 and 0.66, respectively)

Table 6.2 (continued)

References	Sample	Regimen/measure	Procedures	Outcome
Downs, Roberts, Blackmore, Le Souëf, and Jenkins (2006)	$N = 43$ 6–11 yrs ($M = 8$ yrs)	Aerosol and airway clearance treatments (ACT) Caregivers completed 1-wk diaries	Random assignment to control or intervention ("Airways" program; 10-wk pen and paper program completed at home, including information on treatments, decision-making skills, and strategies to overcome barriers to treatment)	Significant group X time interaction in favor of higher adherence to prescribed aerosol treatments in the intervention group ($p < 0.001$) through 12-mo follow-up (but not for prescribed ACT). Also, significant group X time interaction in favor of higher child knowledge of ACT in the intervention group ($p < 0.001$) through 12-mo follow-up.
Hagopian and Thompson (1999)	$N = 1$ 8-yr old male (also mentally retarded and autistic)	Nebulized medications Duration of treatment by direct observation	Withdrawal design (ABAB) A = baseline; B = shaping and positive reinforcement Initial treatment was in an inpatient behavioral unit where the child was also being treated for destructive and aggressive behavior, and then transferred to caretakers in the home	Mean duration was 13.8 s during the first baseline phase, increased to 40 s toward the end of the first treatment phase, dropped to below 10 s in the withdrawal phase, and increased to 37.2 s in the final treatment phase. 14 wks after discharge, adherence was 97.7% (duration of 40 s)
Powers et al. (2005)	$N = 10$ 18 mos.–4 yrs	Dietary intake 7-day food diaries and 24-hr recall (parent report)	Random assignment to behavioral and nutrition (BEH; 6 individual sessions including nutritional and behavior management skill training) or usual/standard care control condition (CTL)	BEH group had significantly higher caloric intake and this was replicated with the 5 patients originally in the CTL who crossed over to BEH. Also, patients receiving BEH met or exceeded normal weight and height velocities.

Table 6.2 (continued)

References	Sample	Regimen/measure	Procedures	Outcome
Stark, Miller, Plienes, and Drabman (1987)	$N = 1$ 11-yr-old female	Chest physiotherapy Patient report with reliability checks by mother	AB case study: A = baseline, B = contracting with gradual fading of rewards Baseline and initial treatment in the hospital and then treatment at home	During 23 days of baseline, patient met goal of 3 treatments per day only once After contracting introduced, patient met goal of 3 treatments per day on all but one day through 9 wks of follow-up
Stark, Mackner, Kessler, Opipari, and Quittner (2002)	$N = 44$ 3–12 yrs ($M = 7.5$ yrs)	Dietary calcium intake Weighed food diaries completed by parents	One-group, pre-posttest design. Parents and children participated in a behavioral intervention, 7 sessions over 9 wks (included dietary information and behavior management strategies, such as differential attention, contingency management, and shaping).	Significant increase in calcium intake from pre- ($M = 1006$ mg) to posttest ($M = 1467$; $p < 0.001$); 12-mo follow-up data for 15 participants showed maintenance of gains
Stark et al. (2003)	$N = 7$ 6–12 yrs ($M = 10$ yrs)	Caloric intake Diet diaries completed by parents	Random assignment to nutrition education (NE; $n = 4$) or behavioral intervention (BI; $n = 3$; nutrition plus behavior management strategies, such as differential attention, contingency management, and shaping) Multiple baseline design to evaluate caloric intake across meals.	Participants in the BI group had a greater increase in daily caloric intake ($M = 1036$ cal/day) and weight gain ($M = 1.42$ kg) than those in the NE group ($M = 408$ cal/day; 0.78 kg) and maintained caloric intake gains at 24-mo follow-up. Multiple baseline showed increases in caloric intake for each meal after introduction of treatment, but to a greater degree for the BI group

Table 6.2 (continued)

Diabetes

References	Sample	Regimen/measure	Procedures	Outcome
Brown et al. (1997)	$N = 59$ 8–16 yrs	Parent report (diabetes self-care questionnaire, rating child's motivation to manage blood glucose testing, taking insulin, and following diet)	Random assignment to experimental group ("Packy & Marlon," a diabetes-related video game emphasizing self-care skills and knowledge) or control group (nondiabetes related video game). All participants played the video games in their homes over a 6-mo period and were given a game system.	Participants in the experimental group showed significantly higher gains in self-care scores at 6-mo follow-up ($p < 0.003$). No differences on HbA_{1c} levels.
Carney, Schechter, and Davis (1983)	$N = 3$ 10–14 yrs	Blood glucose testing Patient records and used testing strips Ghb levels	Multiple baseline across subjects with baseline followed by point system exchanged for money and special activities	All 3 patients showed improvement in % of tests performed with 2 patients improving from <5% in baseline to 87 and 93% after treatment. Gains were maintained at 4 mo follow-up. Ghb levels improved from baseline (10.1, 15.2, and 9.1%) to follow-up (9.4, 11.7, and 6.0%)
Ellis et al. (2005)	$N = 127$ 10–17 yrs	Insulin use, diet, and blood glucose testing by 24-recall interview (with patients) Blood glucose by electronic monitor (glucometer)	Random assignment to standard care or multisystemic therapy (MST). MST is an intensive home- and community-based family therapy approach, which includes a variety of interventions that can be selected including	Significant improvement in the frequency of blood glucose testing (24-hr recall and glucometer) in the MST group vs. standard care group No significant difference between groups in metabolic control, insulin or dietary adherence, and ER visits

Table 6.2 (continued)

References	Sample	Regimen/measure	Procedures	Outcome
			cognitive-behavioral therapy; parent training, family therapy, enlisting support from school personnel and peers, and working with health-care team (mean length of MST was 5.7 mos)	Youth in MST groups showed significant reductions in hospital admissions
Ellis et al. (2007)	$N = 127$ 10–17 yrs	Blood glucose testing Electronic monitor (glucometer)	Random assignment to standard care or multisystemic therapy (MST). MST is an intensive home- and community-based family therapy approach, which includes a variety of interventions that can be selected including cognitive-behavioral therapy; parent training, family therapy, enlisting support from school personnel and peers, and working with health-care team (mean length of MST was 5.7 months).	Significant improvement in the frequency of blood glucose testing in the MST group vs. standard care group. Trend for youths receiving MST to show greater improvements in metabolic control. For youths in the MST group from single-parent families, there was a significant improvement in metabolic control. No differences in primary caregiver support for diabetes. Youth in two-parent families did report significant increase in secondary caregiver support vs. controls in two-parent families.

Table 6.2 (continued)

References	Sample	Regimen/measure	Procedures	Outcome
Epstein et al., (1981)	$N = 17$ 6–16 yrs	Urine glucose testing Direct observation	Random assignment to practice condition (patients tested 20 prepared samples, but not informed of results) or feedback condition (patients tested samples and given feedback about accuracy)	Mean number of correct urine glucose estimations was significantly higher for feedback (7.2) vs. practice (3.8) conditions posttraining
Gilbert et al. (1982)	$N = 28$ 6–9 yrs	Insulin injections (Direct observations (observers rating pass/fail on 27 items related to insulin injection)	Random assignment to treatment or control group; treatment group shown peer-modeling film depicting successful self-injection; control group shown nutrition film	Older girls viewing peer-modeling film showed greater self-injection skill compared to older girls viewing the control film
Gross (1983)	$N = 4$ 10–12 yrs	Urine testing Patient report (with parent counts of used test tablets as a reliability check; overall agreement averaged 80%)	Multiple baseline across subjects; following baseline, patients received self-management training and developed a behavioral contract with parents	Frequency of urine testing improved for all patients; mean % of days urine testing was done 4 times per day increased from 9% during baseline to 74% during self-management condition; at 2- and 4-wk follow-up, frequency of testing dropped for 2 of 4 patients
Gross, Magalnick, and Richardson (1985)	$N = 14$ 9–13 yrs	Diet, glucose testing, and insulin injections Parental report	Random assignment to control or experimental group (included multiple-baseline design) Self-management training (negotiating, contracting, etc.)	Improvements noted in specific adherence behaviors for experimental group patients. No difference in metabolic control between groups.

Table 6.2   (continued)

References	Sample	Regimen/measure	Procedures	Outcome
Howe et al. (2005)	$N = 75$ 2.8–16.9 yrs ($M = 12.4$ yrs)	Diet, exercise, blood glucose monitoring, ketones testing and management Clinician ratings (yes or no for 11 items)	Random assignment to standard care (SC), education (ED; single education session with a nurse focusing on diabetes management), or education + telephone case management (ED + ECM: education session + weekly phone calls to monitor management and behavior management skills with parents)	Adherence scores (% items scored as "yes") significantly higher at 6-mo follow-up in the ED + TCM group (improved by 24% from baseline) vs. the SC group (improved by 2%; $p = 0.0002$)
Kumar, Wentzell, Mikkelsen, Pentland, and Laffel (2004)	$N = 40$ 8–18 yrs	Blood glucose testing Electronic monitoring	Random assignment to control or experimental group. Both groups received PDA with wireless modem and diabetes management software. Experimental group also received a game which allowed them to predict blood glucose levels.	Over the 4-wk trial, significantly more participants in the experimental group (78%) checked blood glucose levels a median of four or more times daily vs. the control group (68%). No significant differences in glycemic control (HbA1C) at ~4-mo follow-up.
Laffel et al. (2003)	$N = 105$ 8–17 yrs ($M = 12$ yrs)	Diet, glucose testing, and insulin injections Clinician rating	Random assignment to standard care (SC) group or family-focused teamwork (TW) group (negotiating sharing of responsibility for diabetes management, communicating, avoiding conflicts, and problem solving)	No significant difference in blood glucose monitoring at 1-year follow-up; A1c levels significantly different ($p < 0.05$) with no deterioration in the TW group from baseline levels; families in the TW group maintained or increased family involvement in diabetes management more than those in SC group (30% vs. 14%; $p = 0.05$)

Table 6.2 (continued)

References	Sample	Regimen/measure	Procedures	Outcome
Lawson, Cohen, Richardson, and Orrbine (2005)	$N = 46$ 13–17 yrs ($M = 15$ yrs)	Diet, glucose testing, and insulin injections Self-report (1–9 point Likert scale, with higher value for higher adherence) Electronic monitoring (glucometer) for glucose testing	Random assignment to standard care or standard care plus weekly telephone contact by a diabetes nurse educator over 6 mos (discussed blood glucose test results and insulin dosing)	During the intervention and at 3-mo follow-up, no significant adherence differences between groups. At 6-mo follow-up, significantly higher ratings for only dietary adherence in the intervention group ($M = 5.7$) vs. the standard care group ($M = 5$; $p = 0.02$).
Lowe and Lutzker (1979)	$N = 1$ 9 yrs	Urine testing, diet, and foot care Direct observation by parent and sibling	Multiple baseline across behaviors Education and token system	Education effective in improving dietary adherence; token system increased adherence to urine testing (from baseline mean of 16 to 97%) and foot care (from baseline mean of 72 to 100%)
Méndez and Beléndez (1997)	$N = 37$ 11–18 yrs ($M = 13$ yrs)	Blood glucose testing Patient report	Quasi-experimental pretest–posttest design. Assignment to control (usual care) or experimental group (12 group sessions, including education about diabetes, stress management, social skills, and blood glucose testing)	Blood glucose testing skills and frequency were significantly higher at immediate posttest for the experimental group (p's < 0.02), but frequency was not significantly different at 13-mo follow-up.

Table 6.2 (continued)

References	Sample	Regimen/measure	Procedures	Outcome
Satin et al. (1989)	$N = 32$ ($M = 14.6$ yrs)	Insulin use Urine glucose testing Diet Exercise Parental ratings of self-care (1 = "very careful" to 5 = "careless") Ghb levels Attitudes toward teenage with diabetes scales Family environment scale	Random assignment to one of three groups: Gr 1: patients and parents met for 6 weekly sessions to discuss diabetes and management; Gr 2: identical to Gr 1 plus included a parent simulation of diabetes regimen; or Gr 3: control group	No significant differences between groups in self-care ratings Significant decrease in Ghb levels at 6-wk postintervention for Gr 2 vs. Gr 3 Significant difference in attitudes toward teenager with diabetes (more positive) for Grs 1 and 2
Schafer, Glasgow, and McCaul (1982)	$N = 3$ 16–18 yrs	Urine glucose testing, insulin use, exercise Wearing diabetic information bracelet and blood glucose testing Assessed by patient self-monitoring records	Multiple baseline across behaviors design with baseline followed by goal setting and (if needed) contingency contracting conditions	Goal setting alone effective in improving adherence to wearing (information), exercise, and urine testing for subject 1 and for urine testing and exercise for subject 2; goal setting plus contracting improved adherence to insulin use for subject 2; nothing effective for subject 3 who was experiencing severe family problems
Silverman, Hains, Davies, and Parton (2003)	$N = 6$ 11–19 yrs	Glucose testing, insulin injections, exercise, and diet 24-hr recall (used patient data only) Electronic monitoring (glucometer) Diabetes-related stress	Multiple baseline across participants with baseline followed by cognitive-behavioral intervention (cognitive restructuring and problem solving)	Intervention improved at least one self-care behavior for 5 of 6 participants; diabetes-related stress reduced in 2 participants

Table 6.2 (continued)

References	Sample	Regimen/measure	Procedures	Outcome
Snyder (1987)	$N = 1$ 14 yrs	Insulin use Urine glucose testing Diet Patient self-monitoring records with independent checks by mother and school nurse	Quasiexperimental single-subject design Following self-monitoring baseline, patient exposed to self-monitoring plus monetary incentives and then to an additional condition involving hospitalization contingent on hypo- or hyperglycemic episodes for 36 hr in a private room with no TV, visitors, books, and minimal staff interaction Behavioral contracting and communication/conflict resolution training were also implemented for antisocial behavior and mother–child conflict	Mean number of diabetes self-care activities performed was 5.6 during self-monitoring baseline, 6.3 during self-monitoring + reinforcement, and 8.5 during self-monitoring + reinforcement + punishment; 1-mo follow-up showed maintenance of gains Also, decreases in antisocial behavior and conflicts and increases in school attendance noted However, anecdotal reports at 6-mo posttreatment indicated deterioration of gains with patient hospitalized for drug abuse
Wysocki, Green, and Huxtable (1989)	$N = 42$ ($M = 14$ yrs)	Blood-glucose testing Insulin use Diet Exercise Electronic monitoring (glucometer)	30 patients randomly assigned to meter-alone (MA) or meter-plus-contract (MC) groups. Remaining 12 patients in conventional-therapy (CT) control group	By 8th wk, MC Gr. had significantly higher frequency of glucose testing No differences in overall adherence, Ghb levels, or patient/parent attitudes and adjustment to diabetes

Table 6.2 (continued)

References	Sample	Regimen/measure	Procedures	Outcome
		24-hr recall patient and parent interviews Ghb levels Attitudes toward diabetes and diabetes adjustment scales	MA Gr. patients earned money for bringing meters to clinic. MC Gr. patients earned money contingent on glucose-testing frequency	
Wysocki et al. (2006)	$N = 104$ 11–16 yrs	Insulin use, blood glucose testing, diet, exercise, and managing hypoglycemia by structured interview (patient and parent scores combined)	Random assignment to standard care (SC), educational support (ES; 12 multifamily meetings for diabetes education and support), or behavioral family systems therapy for diabetes (BFST-D; 12 sessions focusing on problem-solving, communication, cognitive restructuring, and family therapy). The BFST-D was revised for this study to also include having families target two or more diabetes-related problems, behavioral contracting training, use of self-monitoring of blood glucose data, and parents simulating living with diabetes for 1 wk.	Main effect of group and the group X time interaction showed no significant differences on adherence BFST-D did yield significant improvements (or fewer declines) for youth with higher baseline HbA1c levels vs. the other groups Main effect of group and the group X time interaction showed no significant differences on metabolic control Improvements in metabolic control were significantly greater for those with higher baseline HbA1c for the BFST-D and ES groups vs. SC group Diabetes responsibility and conflict scores significantly improved for the BFST-D vs. the other groups Parental–adolescent relationship scores (conflict, extreme belief, family structure) did not differ between the groups

Table 6.2 (continued)

References	Sample	Regimen/measure	Procedures	Outcome
		Gastrointestinal disorders		
Stark et al. (2005a)	$N = 32$ with inflammatory bowel disease 5–12 yrs	Calcium intake Weighed food diaries kept by parents	Random assignment to enhanced standard of care (ESC: 3 sessions over 8 wks and given nutritional information and handouts) or behavioral intervention (BI: 6 sessions over 8 wks and given nutritional information and handouts + parents and children given behavior management strategies shaping, sticker chart, home-based rewards, and problem solving to reduce barriers)	Significant condition and time interaction with children in the BI group achieving higher calcium intake levels vs. ESC group (M increase 984 mg/Ca/day vs. 274 mg/Ca/day; $p < 0.001$); also significantly higher % of children in the BI group reached the goal of 1500 mg/Ca/day vs. ESC group (81% vs. 19%; $p < 0.001$)
		Hemophilia		
Gilbert and Varni (1988)	$N = 1$ 10 yrs	Factor replacement therapy Observation of patient completing factor replacement using a behavior checklist	Case study with baseline, treatment and 4-and-half-mos follow-up measures obtained; following baseline, nurse modeled correct performance of factor replacement skills, had patient rehearse skills, gave corrective feedback as needed, and praised for correct performance	Mean adherence to proper technique ranged from 0 to 89% across factor replacement behavioral categories during baseline; this range improved to 83–98% during treatment and 100% during follow-up

Table 6.2 (continued)

References	Sample	Regimen/measure	Procedures	Outcome
Greenan-Fowler, Powell, and Varni (1987)	$N = 10$ 8–15 yrs	Home physical therapy program Patient report (written records) and attendance at exercise class	One group, repeated measures quasi-experimental design; following baseline, patients and parents were exposed to behavior management training (shaping, token system, etc.) for 12 wks; follow-up assessments were done at 3, 6, and 9 mos posttreatment	Adherence to exercises significantly higher during treatment (mean = 96%), 3-mo (mean = 91%), and 6-mo (mean = 85%) follow-up compared to baseline (mean = 55%), but not at 9-mo follow-up (mean = 63%); session attendance did not vary significantly between measurement periods
Sergis-Davenport and Varni (1983)	$N = 12$ parents	Factor replacement therapy Direct observation using a behavioral checklist	Nonrandom assignment to treatment or control group; parents in treatment group were given systematic training in factor replacement therapy in 2 hr weekly visits over a 4- to 8-wk period; control group parents did not receive special training	Mean % of correct performance in factor replacement skills increased significantly from 15% at baseline to 92% during intervention for treatment-group parents; percentages significantly higher for treatment vs. control group at follow-up

HIV

References	Sample	Regimen/measure	Procedures	Outcome
Berrien, Salazar, Reynolds, and McKay (2004)	$N = 37$ 1.5–20 yrs ($M = 10$ yrs)	Medications (antiretroviral therapy) Pharmacy refills (scored from 0 to 3, where 0 = "never refilled" to 3 = "monthly refill")	Random assignment to control (education and a single home visit if necessary) or intervention group (8 home visits over a 3-mo period by a nurse with enhanced education using a comic book and video, addressing barriers to	Adherence by pharmacy refill was significantly higher in the intervention group ($M = 2.7$) vs. the control group (1.7; $p = 0.002$). No significant differences on self-reported adherence, CD4 count, or viral load.

Table 6.2 (continued)

References	Sample	Regimen/measure	Procedures	Outcome
		Self-report (by questionnaire, with perfect score = 37)	adherence, tracking medication use with a notebook and stickers, and receiving prizes for tracking adherence)	No significant pre-posttest differences on adherence (M's = 98 to 97%). Significant improvement in viral load, pre- to posttest.
Ellis, Naar-King, Cunningham, and Secord (2006)	$N = 19$ 20 mos–16 yrs ($M = 11$ yrs)	Medications Caregiver report (rated on 0–100%, with 100% = "perfect adherence" during the previous month)	Retrospective chart review on families who received in-home multisystemic therapy over an average of 7 mos (intensive and individualized treatment involving cognitive-behavioral therapy, parent training, behavioral family systems therapy, and communication skills training techniques)	
Garvie et al., (2007)	$N = 23$ 4–22 yrs	Highly active antiretroviral therapy (HAART) by pharmacy pill counts	Retrospective chart review of 23 patients clinically referred for pill-swallowing problems. Modeling and shaping (starting with small pieces of candy and progressing to placebo pills the size of prescribed medications) used to teach pill swallowing	Adherence increased by a median of 9.8% Percentage of patients showing no evidence of immune suppression increased from 50% at baseline to 81.8% at ~6 mos.
Shingadia et al. (2000)	$N = 17$ 1.25–11.8 yrs (Mdn = 2.9 yrs)	HAART medications Physician or nurse rating	Retrospective chart review of children who received gastrostomy tube (GT) placement for medication administration	In the year before GT placement, "good adherence" recorded in 6 patients (35%), 7 were nonadherent (41%), and in 4 patients (23%) adherence not documented; all 17 (100%) were noted to be adherent after GT placement

Table 6.2 (continued)

Renal

References	Sample	Regimen/measure	Procedures	Outcome
Beck et al. (1980)	$N = 21$ 3–20 yrs ($M = 14.6$ yrs)	Immunosuppressive drugs, posttransplant. Pill counts	One-group, pre-post test design Baseline assessment followed by 6 mos of physician counseling and regimen simplification when feasible	Initially 9 of 21 were nonadherent (43%); 4 of these 9 remained nonadherent, while 5 were adherent after 6 mos of physician counseling
Carton and Schweitzer (1996)	$N = 1$ 10 yrs	Hemodialysis Direct observation	ABAB single-subject design. Baseline followed by token system, which was withdrawn, reinstated, and faded	Nonadherence to hemodialysis reduced with token system and worsened when the token system was withdrawn; nonadherence remained low at 3- and 6-mofollow-up
Fennell, Foulkes, and Boggs (1994)	$N = 29$ 5–18 yrs ($M = 12$ yrs)	Immunosuppressive medications, posttransplant Pill counts (azathioprine and prednisone) Blood assay (cyclosporine)	Participants matched by age and gender and assigned to control group (standard care) or experimental group (educational booklet, 10-minute videotape, medication calendar, and reward system)	Adherence significantly better with prednisone only for experimental group vs. control group, at 4–6 wks and 8–12 wks follow-up
Magrab and Papadopoulou (1977)	$N = 4$	Dietary regimen Weight, blood and urine tests (nitrogen and potassium levels)	Reversal design Baseline and token system conditions	Weight gain acceptable during treatment vs. baseline. Some improvements in nitrogen and potassium levels for two children.

Table 6.2 (continued)

Rheumatic diseases

References	Sample	Regimen/measure	Procedures	Outcome
Pieper et al., (1989)	$N = 3$ 11–18 yrs 2 patients with systemic lupus erythematosus and 1 with dermatomyositis	Medications Pill counts	Multiple baseline across subjects. Following baseline, patients and parents given instructions in clinic about medications, adherence, and monitoring/reinforcement strategies	Because over- as well as underdosing occurred, patients classified as adherent if pill counts indicated 80–120% of doses were taken. The mean % of pill counts in acceptable range was baseline = 38, 7, and 33%; intervention = 89, 67, and 88%; 6-month follow-up = 100% for all patients; and 12-month follow-up = 67% for 2 patients.
Rapoff et al., (1984)	$N = 1$ 7 yrs JRA	Medications, splints, and prone lying exercise Parent observations with inter-observer reliability checks in home (mean agreement = 94% for medications and 100% for splints and prone lying)	Multiple baseline across behaviors with 10-wk follow-up; token system introduced following baseline	Baseline mean adherence was 59% for medications, 0% for splints and prone lying exercise; improved to 95, 77, and 71%, respectively during treatment and 90, 91, and 80%, respectively, at 10-wk follow-up
Rapoff et al., (1988a)	$N = 1$ 14 yrs JRA	Medications Pill counts	Single-subject withdrawal design. Following baseline, regimen simplified (q.i.d to t.i.d); token system in the home for 10 wks, then withdrawn for 7 wks, reinstated for 7 wks, and then maintenance phase for 8 wks	Mean adherence levels by condition were baseline = 44%; simplified regimen = 59%; token system = 100%; withdrawal of token system = 77%; token system reinstated = 99%; maintenance phase = 92%; and 9-month follow-up = 97%.

Table 6.2 (continued)

References	Sample	Regimen/measure	Procedures	Outcome
			(where token system reintroduced if adherence was <80% for 2 consecutive wks). Token system then completely withdrawn	Less disease activity evident during simplified regimen and token system phases.
Rapoff et al., (1988b)	N = 3 3, 10, and 13 yrs JRA	Medications Pill counts	Multiple baseline across subjects design. Following baseline, treatment introduced across participants in a time-staggered fashion and involved a single home visit where information was reviewed about type and purpose of medications prescribed, the importance of consistent adherence, how to prevent medication side effects, and monitoring of adherence and positive feedback	By visual inspection, adherence improved for the 10-and 3-yr old participants from mean baseline levels of 38 and 54%, respectively, to 97 and 92%, respectively, during intervention; at 4-mo follow-up mean adherence levels were 56 and 89%, respectively, for these participants. Adherence increased only slightly for the 13-yr-old participant, averaging 44% at baseline and 49% during intervention; at 4-mo follow-up, adherence dropped to an average of 24%.
Rapoff et al. (2002)	N = 34 2–16 yrs Newly diagnosed with JRA	Medications Electronic monitor (MEMS)	Random assignment to education/behavioral intervention or education only control group. Procedures for both groups introduced during 30-min clinic visit by the clinic	Over the 52-wk period of study, participants in the education/behavioral group showed significant better overall mean adherence than the controls (77.7% vs. 56.9%).

Table 6.2 (continued)

References	Sample	Regimen/measure	Procedures	Outcome
			nurse, and then the nurse phoned participants every 2 wks for 2 months and then monthly for 10 mos.	No significant differences between groups on measures of disease activity (active joint counts, morning stiffness, global disease severity, or functional limitations).
			Audio-visual programs and handouts used with both groups. Education group received information about types of JRA, signs and symptoms, and treatments,	
			Education/behavioral group received information identical to control group plus strategies for maintaining adherence, such as cueing, monitoring, positive reinforcement, and discipline.	
Stark et al. (2005b)	$N = 49$ 4–10 yrs	Calcium (Ca) intake Weighed food diaries by parents	Random assignment to enhanced standard of care (ESC; 3 sessions over 8 wks and given nutritional information and handouts) or behavioral intervention (BI; 6 sessions over 8 wks and given nutritional information and handouts + parents and children given	Significant group by time interaction with children in the BI group achieving a greater increase in Ca intake vs. those in ESC group ($M = 829$ mg/Ca/day vs. 320 mg/Ca/day; $p < 0.001$); 92% of children in BI group achieved treatment goal of 1500 mg/Ca/day vs. 17% in ESC group ($p < 0.001$).

Table 6.2 (continued)

References	Sample	Regimen/measure	Procedures	Outcome
			behavior management strategies shaping, sticker chart, home-based rewards, and problem solving to reduce barriers)	
Seizures				
Dawson and Jamieson (1971)	N = 30 6 mos–12 yrs	Medications Blood assays over a 6-mo period	One-group pre- and posttest quasi-experimental design; after initial blood levels were obtained, patients were monitored monthly by assays with parental and patient knowledge	At the beginning of the study, only 25% of sample had therapeutic blood levels and this increased to 80% by the end of study.
Sickle cell disease				
Berkovitch et al. (1998)	N = 45 9 mos–7 yrs (M = 3 yrs)	Prophylactic penicillin Electronic monitor (MEMS)	Random assignment to intervention group (slide show about pathogenesis of sickle cell disease, complications, and importance of therapy; stickers and calendar to track adherence; and weekly phone calls by social worker) or control group	Mean adherence for the intervention group was 66% at baseline and 79% at 2-mo follow-up vs. 69 and 66%, respectively, for the control group (not significantly different). Loss of 13 participants due to change to tablet from liquid preparation (because MEMS device was damaged by liquid medications and children could not swallow tablets).

McDonald, & Yao, 2008). At least two meta-analyses have examined the relative effectiveness of adherence interventions across many patient conditions and adherence measures (Peterson, Takiya, & Finley, 2003; Roter et al., 1998). The Peterson et al. (2003) meta-analysis concluded that despite being intensive and complex, the effect sizes for adherence interventions were generally small. In contrast, the Roter et al. (1998) meta-analysis found that overall effect sizes for interventions ranged from small to large. Roter and colleagues also concluded that combined-type interventions (e.g., educational and behavioral) were more effective than single-type interventions. This difference in conclusions may be because Roter et al. (1998) included both randomized and nonrandomized studies, whereas Peterson et al. (2003) included only randomized clinical trials. Both meta-analyses had notable limitations, including combining acute and chronic illnesses, as well as adult- and child-focused interventions. The Peterson et al. (2003) meta-analysis also included psychiatric illnesses.

Meta-Analysis of Adherence Interventions for Acute Pediatric Diseases

One meta-analysis has been published on interventions to promote adherence to medications for otitis media and streptococcal pharyngitis in children (Wu & Roberts, 2008). A total of 12 studies were included in the meta-analysis, which included an average sample size of 150 (range = 30–512) and a sample composition of 52.4% Caucasians. Mean effect sizes (weighted by sample size) ranged from small to large across types of interventions, with the highest effect size for combined educational and behavioral interventions ($d = 1.33$, 95% confidence interval (CI) = $0.94 - 1.72$) and a small to medium effect size in favor of the control group for educational interventions ($d = -0.42$, CI = $-0.60 - 0.23$). Mean weighted ES ranged from a small to medium effect for indirect measures of adherence (e.g., pill counts) in favor of the treatment group ($d = 0.49$, CI = $0.36 - 0.63$) to a small to medium effect for direct measures (e.g., urine assay) in favor of the control group ($d = -0.46$, CI = $-0.66 - 0.25$). Secondary outcomes (illness remission or appointment keeping) were not significantly affected by adherence interventions.

Meta-Analyses of Adherence Interventions for Chronic Pediatric Diseases

Two meta-analyses on interventions to promote adherence to regimens for chronic pediatric disease could be located for this review (Graves, Roberts, Rapoff, & Boyer, in press; Kahana, Drotar, & Frazier, 2008). The first meta-analysis includes 70 studies with a mean sample age of 10.24 years (range 2–15 years) and a sample composition of 82% Caucasians (Kahana et al., 2008). The number of studies by disease is as follows: 32 (45.7%) asthma, 16 (22.9%) diabetes, 10 (14.3%) cystic fibrosis, 2 each with JRA and obesity (2.9% respectively), and one each for hemodialysis, hemophilia, HIV, IBD, PKU, seizures, sickle cell disease, and tuberculosis (1.4% each). Of the 70 studies, 29 (41.4%) were identified as randomized controlled trials and 42 (60%) reported effect sized based on an experimental versus control group design, while 19 (27.1%) reported effect size based on pre-post differences and another 9 (12.9%) reported both.

The mean weighted (by sample size) effect size across all adherence measures was in the small to medium range ($d = 0.34$, CI $= 0.34 - 0.73$). Because there was significant heterogeneity across adherence outcomes, the authors examined potential moderators (Kahana et al., 2008). Outcomes differed by type of intervention, as follows: behavioral ($d = 0.54$, CI $= 0.34 - 0.73$), multicomponent ($d = 0.52$, CI $= 0.45 - 0.57$), psychosocial ($d = 0.44$, CI $= 0.23 - 0.65$), educational ($d = 0.16$, CI $= 0.10 - 0.22$), and technology-based ($d = 0.08$, CI $= - 0.09 - 0.25$). Mean weighted effect sizes were different depending on the regimen component that was targeted, with self-management, self-care behaviors, dietary change, and exercise-environmental changes yielding small to medium effect sizes (d's ranging from 0.47 to 0.52), while medications yielded small effect sizes ($d = 0.20$). Mean weighted effect sizes were also different depending on disease type, with medium to large for cystic fibrosis ($d = 0.74$), medium for miscellaneous disorders ($d = 0.54$), small to medium for diabetes ($d = 0.38$), and small for asthma ($d = 0.23$). Studies that combined pre-post and experimental versus control group designs produced medium to large effect sizes ($d = 0.65$), pre-post only designs produced small to medium effect sizes ($d = 0.42$), and experimental versus control group designs produced a small effect size ($d = 0.23$). Effect sizes were also found to diminish over time as follows: 0–6 month follow-up $d = 0.63$ (CI $= 0.46 - 0.80$); 7–12 months $d = 0.24$ (CI $= 0.06 - 0.42$); and >12 months $d = -0.50$ (CI $= -1.15 - 0.15$). The authors' conclusion was that behavioral and multicomponent interventions are "relatively potent" in enhancing adherence to regimens for chronic pediatric diseases (Kahana et al., 2008).

The other meta-analysis on adherence interventions for chronic pediatric diseases includes 71 studies, only 19 of which overlap with the Kahana et al. (2008) meta-analysis (Graves et al., in press). It also differs from the Kahana et al. (2008) review in that self-management interventions were not included (as they had gone beyond just targeting adherence) and studies using single-subject designs were included in the Graves et al. meta-analysis. Of the 71 studies, 34 (48.6%) used a comparison group design (e.g., experimental versus control group), 17 (24.3%) used a within-subject group design (one group pre-post design), and 19 (27.1%) used a single-subject design. The mean age of participants in the group design studies was 9.9 years (range $= 2$–15years) and in the single-subject design studies, it was 11 years (range 2–17 years). Of the 22 group design studies, which reported on ethnicity, the percentage of minority group participants averaged 39.1% (range $= 0$–100%) and of the four single-subject design studies reporting on ethnicity, two had no minority participants and two had 100% minority participants. Of the group design studies ($n = 51$), 16 studies involved asthma (31.4%), 15 with type-1 diabetes (29.4%), 5 with CF (9.8%), 3 each with HIV/ AIDS or posttransplant (5.9% each), 2 each with hyperlipidemia, JRA, and sickle cell disease (3.9% each), and one each with epilepsy, hemophilia, and phenylketonuria (2% each). Of the single-subject design studies ($n = 19$), 7 studies involved type-1 diabetes (36.8%), 3 each with JRA and CF (15.8% each), 2 with asthma (10.5%), and one each with epilepsy, lung disease, various rheumatic diseases, and sickle cell (5.3% each). Of the group design studies, the control group was assigned an alternative treatment in 11 studies (32.4%), treatment as usual in 20 studies (58.8%), and waitlist in 3 studies (8.8%). Of the 71 studies, 24 (34%) included follow-up adherence data and 38 (54%) included a direct (A1C, body mass index, or pulmonary function tests) or an indirect health outcome measure (disease activity estimates, health-care utilization, or HRQOL). The weighted (by sample size) mean effect size across all of the adherence outcomes in the group design studies was in the medium range ($d = 0.58$, CI $= 0.51 – 0.65$). The weighted mean effect across all of the single-subject adherence data was in the large range ($d = 1.53$, 95% CI $= 1.07 – 1.98$). Because there was a significant amount of heterogeneity among the effect sizes for the group design studies only, potential moderators were examined for these studies (Graves et al., in press). The studies using a single intervention method had higher mean effect sizes (educational only: $d = 0.56$, behavioral only: $d = 0.51$, organizational only: $d = 0.50$) than the studies with combined educational and behavioral interventions ($d = 0.36$). However, a follow-up analysis of between-group differences was not significant. Group design studies using a waitlist design had a significantly stronger mean effect size ($d = 1.09$) than those using an alternative treatment ($d = 0.43$) or treatment as usual ($d = 0.56$). There was also some homogeneity when the data were organized by outcome type. The effect sizes were homogeneous within direct (i.e., blood/ urine tests) and indirect (i.e., pill count and electronic monitoring) measures, but not within the subjective measures (i.e., child and parent report). When direct measures are used to measure adherence, the mean effect size ($d = 0.20$, CI $= -0.08 – 0.48$) suggests that adherence interventions are not successful at increasing adherence. Mean effect sizes were highest for group design studies involving patients with asthma ($d = 0.58$), followed by other illnesses combined ($d = 0.57$), and diabetes (0.42).

The weighted mean effect size across all of the follow-up adherence data in the group design studies was in the medium range ($d = 0.48$, CI $= 0.28 – 0.69$). The weighted mean effect size of the single-subject follow-up adherence data was in the large range ($d = 1.44$, CI $= 0.99 – 1.89$). Unlike the effect sizes from the single-subject studies, there was a significant amount of heterogeneity in effect sizes for the group design studies and moderators were examined. One significant moderator was regimen type and the strongest follow-up mean effect size was in adherence to diet ($d = 0.86$, CI $= 0.35 – 1.38$), followed by exercise ($d = 0.79$, CI $= 0.19 – 1.38$), medications ($d = 0.47$, CI $= 0.09 – 0.85$), and overall disease management ($d = .27$, CI $= 0.03 – 0.51$).

The weighted mean effect size across all of the health outcomes in the group design studies was in the medium range ($d = 0.40$, CI $= 0.31 – 0.50$) and for the single-subject design studies in the large range ($d = 0.74$, CI $= 0.19 - 1.29$). Again, unlike the single-subject effect sizes, there was significant heterogeneity among the group design studies, so moderators were examined. Health outcome measurements from studies using a pre-post design had a stronger mean effect size ($d = 1.27$, CI $= 1.05 - 1.50$) than the studies using a comparison group design ($d = 0.22$, CI $= 0.12 - 0.32$). Additionally, positive health outcomes were stronger in studies focused on children with asthma ($d = 0.86$, CI $= 0.67 - 1.05$) compared to those targeting children with diabetes ($d = 0.29$, CI $= 0.13 - 0.45$) or other diagnoses ($d = 0.24$, CI $= 0.10 - 0.39$). Finally, in contrast to the adherence outcomes, effect sizes for the health outcomes were higher for studies using a combination of educational and behavioral interventions ($d = 0.74$, CI $= 0.55 - 0.94$) while single intervention-type studies had the smallest effect size ($d = 0.16$, CI $= 0.02 - 0.30$). Graves et al. concluded that adherence interventions effectively increase adherence, adherence gains are maintained over time, and they have a positive impact on health outcomes.

Conclusions from the Meta-Analyses

The one meta-analysis of adherence interventions for acute pediatric diseases showed lower effect sizes on adherence, particularly for more direct measures (such as assays) compared to the meta-analyses for chronic pediatric diseases (Wu & Roberts, 2008). The two meta-analyses for chronic pediatric diseases showed that adherence interventions produce small to medium effect sizes and the Graves et al. meta-analysis also showed positive health benefits. Meta-analyses in the adult literature have also shown small to medium effect sizes for adherence interventions and small but significant effects on health outcomes (Peterson et al., 2003; Roter et al., 1998). The two pediatric meta-analyses for chronic diseases also show that single interventions (behavioral, educational, or organizational) can be more beneficial than combined ones, which contradicts other qualitative reviews of the literature (e.g., Rapoff, 1999). They also highlight the importance of the type of research design used to evaluate interventions. Single-subject designs and group designs without a control group produce higher adherence effect sizes. This makes sense with single-subject design studies because there was little variance in the type of intervention used, with almost half of the studies using behavioral techniques alone and most of the other studies using educational and behavioral techniques combined (Graves et al., in press). The single-subject studies also had lower variance with respect to outcome assessment techniques used and the diagnoses of the children in the studies. In addition, those who use single-subject designs pay attention to visual displays of individual patient's data and have to show large effects to convince their colleagues that a change has been made relative to baseline levels (Barlow, Nock, & Hersen, 2009). They may, therefore, employ more powerful behavioral techniques to increase adherence. Alternatively, single-subject design studies that do not show a convincing effect are not likely to be published. Group designs that employ a waitlist control or pre-post design are subjecting adherence interventions to a less stringent test of their efficacy. Whereas, those using an attention placebo or alternative treatment control group have to show that the "active" ingredients of their intervention are more effective than nonspecific factors, like increased attention.

The qualitative review in this chapter and the meta-analyses reviewed document that interventions in pediatric psychology for improving adherence can be effective, particularly for chronic conditions. Once a sufficient corpus of studies are available, disease-specific meta-analyses will be needed which should help increase homogeneity of results. This has been done for educational interventions that target lung function, self-efficacy, and functional limitations for children and adolescents with asthma (Guevara, Wolf, Grum, & Clark, 2003). We also need to continue to demonstrate that improvements in adherence are concomitant with improvements in disease and health outcome. There is room for much improvement as I conclude with recommendations for making such improvements in pediatric medical adherence research.

Top Ten Ways to Advance Pediatric Medical Adherence Research (With Apologies to My Colleagues Who Have Heard Me Present This at Two Different National Meetings)

1. *We need to settle on a standard definition of adherence.* As discussed in Chapter 1, the definition by the World Health Organization retains important elements of the old standby definition by Haynes (1979) and adds language which implies that agreement to follow regimens has been secured from the patient and parents. The definition offered by the World Health Organization defines adherence as "the extent to which a person's behavior – taking medication, following a diet, and/or executing lifestyle changes, corresponds with agreed recommendations from a health care provider" (World Health Organization, 2003, pp. 3–4). If we all use this definition, it may become the standard here in the United States and internationally.

2. *We need to develop standard scores derived from adherence measures and determine cutpoints for classifying people into adherent and nonadherent categories.* In Chapter 4, several adherence scores were recommended by Kastrissios et al. (1996) for medication adherence. For other regimen components other dimensions will be important, such as duration and intensity of exercise. Cutpoints need to be based on data suggesting that a certain minimum level of adherence is necessary to see meaningful therapeutic changes. This is going to vary by disease and regimen types. The old standard of 80% for medication adherence is not sufficient for some regimens, such as the need for 95% or better adherence to antiretroviral medications in the treatment of HIV.

3. *We need to revise, rework, and make adherence theories relevant to pediatrics.* Virtually all of the theories which offer predictions about why patients adhere or fail to adhere to medical regimens have been based on studies with adults. The validity and utility of downward extensions of these models to children

and adolescents needs to be verified. Theories are important in that they influence how studies are designed and how researchers react to and make sense of data obtained from their studies. Clinicians and researchers should be careful in adopting existing theories that fail to adequately address the developmental needs, challenges, and capacities of children of various ages and stages of development. For example, assessing self-efficacy perceptions would be relevant for children after they acquire the necessary language and cognitive facility to make these types of judgments about their capabilities to perform a given action. Before they acquire the necessary prerequisite skills, the self-efficacy judgments of parents or caretakers would seem to be more relevant.

4. *We need to develop reliable, valid, sensitive, and practical self-report measures of adherence.* The more objective measures, such as assays and electronic monitor, can be invasive, expensive, and not available for all regimen components. Soliciting patient and caretaker reports about adherence remains the most direct and practical way to assess adherence in clinical practice. The way questions are posed can affect how willingly and accurately patients and caregivers report about adherence. Framing questions in a nonjudgmental and time-limited fashion will likely yield more honest and useful reports about adherence. Structured telephone interviews appear to be clinically feasible and would limit recall bias. Also, structured interviews allow clinicians to address ongoing concerns and barriers related to adherence that are revealed by patients and caretakers during periodic phone interviews. As reviewed in Chapter 4 (Table 4.2), there are a number of promising self- and caretaker-report instruments. Some of these, however, are rather lengthy, and further work needs to be done to make them shorter without compromising reliability and validity. For example, we have used one item to assess adherence to inhaled steroids by parent or patient report. The parent report item is: "Some parents have trouble reminding their child to use their inhaled steroid. Would you say that in the last 2 weeks your child has. . . .

- Never taken his/her inhaled steroid (0)
- Forgotten to take his/her inhaled steroid at least 4 times a week (1)
- Forgotten to take his/her inhaled steroid 1–3 times a week (2)
- Rarely forgotten to take his/her inhaled steroid (3)
- Never forgotten to take his/her inhaled steroid (4)"

The maximum score is four indicting perfect adherence over the past 2 weeks. We are currently analyzing this and other measures for a sample of children with asthma. This item has been correlated significantly with an electronic monitoring measures of adherence (MDILog), with the parent report one item measure being obtained at the end of the 2-week electronic monitoring ($r = 0.315, p = 0.007, N = 72$). When we split the sample by median age, the correlation was not significant for children ≥ 10 years ($r = 0.21, p = 0.205$) but remained significant for children <10 years ($r = 0.47, p = 0.005$), suggesting that parent reports are more valid for younger children (Lootens, Rapoff, & Belmont, unpublished data)

5. *We need to continue to develop electronic monitor measures of adherence and extend them to regimen components other than medications.* As reviewed in Chapter 4, electronic methods of data collection have been extended to other regimen components. There is also the capability for technology-based data collection methods that can be entered by patients or parents and accessed by researchers and clinician in real time. Data collected by electronic methods can be downloaded and shared with patients and families to enhance adherence (Kamps et al., 2008).

6. *We need to develop and standardize practical measures of disease activity and quality of life.* Pediatric psychologists will need to work with their medical sub-specialty colleagues to determine measure of disease activity relevant to specific acute and chronic diseases. As reviewed in Chapter 4, pediatric psychologists have been very active in developing and validating HRQOL measures with their medical colleagues (Palermo et al., 2008). We need to continue this work because the ultimate goal of adherence enhancement is that patients have less disease activity and a better quality of life.

7. *We need to validate primary and secondary interventions to prevent or minimize anticipated declines in adherence over time.* Most interventions are designed for children who are suspected of being nonadherent to the extent that it compromises their health. *Primary* prevention would focus on patients not yet exhibiting "clinically significant nonadherence" (CSN), which I defined as "inconsistencies in following a particular regimen that may result in compromised health and well-being" (Rapoff, 2000). Strategies for enhancing adherence at the primary level could involve educational, organizational (e.g., simplifying the regimen), and simple behavioral ones (e.g., increased monitoring by providers). *Secondary* prevention would focus on patients for whom CSN has been identified early on in the diseases course or their nonadherence has not yet compromised health and well-being. Strategies for enhancing adherence at the secondary level might include more frequent monitoring of adherence by caregivers, positive social reinforcement, and routine disciple strategies (e.g., time-out for younger children). The role of pediatric psychologists would be to train health-care providers (particularly nurses) to implement primary and secondary interventions and experimentally evaluate the results of these interventions (e.g., Rapoff et al., 2002).

8. *We need to make better use of single-subject design methodology for intervention studies* (Rapoff & Stark, 2008). Although randomized, between-groups, controlled clinical trials (RCTs) are considered the "gold standard" for experimentally evaluating the efficacy of treatments, there is a long tradition in medicine and psychology of investigating the effects of interventions at the individual level using single-subject designs (Barlow et al., 2009). Single-subject designs offer a number of advantages over traditional group designs: (1) they provide flexibility in the choice of independent variables and allow for changes in these over the course of a study (if something is not working, an intervention can be modified and introduced as a new condition); (2) they accommodate for small sample sizes (appropriate for studying rare conditions or smaller sample

sizes available at any one site); (3) they are appropriate when there are ethical objections to withholding treatment; (4) they are better at exposing individual variability in outcome measures; (5) they produce results that are more easily understood by clinicians (who work at the level of individual patients); (6) they have greater potential for attracting busy clinicians to do clinical research; and (7) they are recognized as legitimate designs that can help establish empirically validated treatments and evidence-based practices (Barlow et al., 2009; Rapoff & Stark, 2008). The most common designs are the reversal and multiple baseline designs that can be used when one patient or more (see Barlow et al., 2009 for the authoritative book on single-subject designs).

9. *We need to develop and test innovative adherence promotion strategies and innovative ways to deliver the interventions.* I would suggest that we would better spend our precious time, resources, and funding to develop and test interventions rather than continuing to feed the correlational machine that promises to discover factors that predict adherence (which it does, see Chapter 2) but fails to take the next step of manipulating factors to affect adherence. As this chapter and the previous one have shown, we know a fair amount about which strategies can be effective in enhancing adherence. We are also on the cusp of delivering interventions in attractive and cost-effective ways, such as technology-based programs. Having developed and tested interventions, I know how difficult and time consuming the process can be, but we are setting a good example for those that we mentor by investing the efforts in enhancing adherence.

10. *We must conduct multisite, randomized controlled adherence intervention trials.* Our medical colleagues have been doing this for many years to develop new drugs and test other medical interventions. Those of us who serve on advisory panels or study sections should lobby for greater funding of multisite studies. The National Institutes of Health allow multiple principal investigators which should help encourage multisite studies. By joining together, we can problem solve about adherence promotion strategies and ways to deliver them and increase our sample sizes needed to adequately power intervention studies.

The Inflated Importance of Adherence

What a paradoxical way to end a book that has emphasized the importance of adherence in improving the health and well-being of children. There are, however, broader psychosocial and medical contexts to consider. *Patient nonadherence may be part of a mosaic of patient and family struggles.* Medical adherence problems may be symptomatic or exist concurrently with patient and/or family dysfunction. For example, a depressed adolescent who has a chronic disease may not have the energy and coping resources to adequately adhere to a complicated medical regimen. These psychological problems need to be addressed by competent mental health personnel who have extensive experience working with patients and families in pediatric settings.

Additionally, *the outcome of medical treatment does not solely depend on adherence*. There are other factors to consider. Subtherapeutic drug assays may reflect low adherence, but can also be due to inadequate dosing, pharmacokinetic variations in drug metabolism, and interactions with other drugs. Health-care providers also have to address health-care disparities for minority children and adolescents. For example, African-American children with asthma living in urban areas have been undermedicated according to nationally recognized treatment guidelines (Eggleston et al., 1998; Halterman et al., 2002). However, the overall message of this book is still relevant. *When confronted with less than adequate outcomes in the treatment of acute and chronic diseases, a reasonable beginning is to investigate the contribution of patient adherenc*e.

References

Aaronson, N. K. (1989). Quality of life assessment in clinical trials: Methodologic issues. *Controlled Clinical Trials, 10*, 1955–2085.

Achenbach, T. M., McConaughy, S. H., & Howell, C. T. (1987). Child/adolescent behavioral and emotional problems: Implications of cross-informant correlations for situational specificity. *Psychological Bulletin, 101*, 213–232.

Achenbach, T. M., & Rescorla, L. A. (2001). *Manual for ASEBA school-age forms & profiles.* Burlington, VT: University of Vermont, Research Center for Children, Youth, & Families.

Adams, C. D., Dreyer, M. L., Dinakar, C., & Portnoy, J. M. (2004). Pediatric asthma: A look at adherence from the patient and family perspective. *Current Allergy & Asthma Reports, 4*, 425–432.

Ajzen, I. (1991). The theory of planned behavior. *Organizational Behavior and Human Decision Processes, 50*, 179–211.

Ajzen, I., & Fishbein, M. (1977). Attitude-behavior relations: A theoretical analysis and review of empirical research. *Psychological Bulletin, 84*, 888–918.

Allen, K. D., & Warzak, W. J. (2000). The problem of parental nonadherence in clinical behavior analysis: Effective treatment is not enough. *Journal of Applied Behavior Analysis, 33*, 373–391.

American Psychiatric Association. (1994). *Diagnostic and statistical manual of mental disorders* (4th ed.). Washington, DC: Author

Anastasia, A. (1988). *Psychological testing* (6th ed.). New York: Macmillan.

Anderson, B., Ho, J., Brackett, J., Finkelstein, D., & Laffel, L. (1997). Parental involvement in diabetes management tasks: Relationships to blood glucose monitoring adherence and metabolic control in young adolescents with insulin-dependent diabetes mellitus. *Journal of Pediatrics, 130*, 257–265.

Anderson, B. J., Auslander, W. F., Jung, D. C., Miller, J. P., & Santiago, J. V. (1990). Assessing family sharing of diabetes responsibilities. *Journal of Pediatric Psychology, 15*, 477–492.

Anderson, C. M., Hawkins, R. P., & Scotti, J. R. (1997). Private events in behavior analysis: Conceptual basis and clinical relevance. *Behavior Therapy, 28*, 157–179.

Anson, O., Weizman, Z., & Zeevi, N. (1990). Celiac disease: Parental knowledge and attitudes of dietary compliance. *Pediatrics, 85*, 98–103.

April, K. T., Feldman, D. E., Zunzunegui, M. V., & Duffy, C. M. (2008). Association between perceived treatment adherence and health-related quality of life in children with juvenile idiopathic arthritis: Perspectives of both parents and children. *Patient Preference and Adherence, 2*, 121–128.

Apter, A. J., Tor, M., & Feldman, H. I. (2001). Testing the reliability of old and new features of a new electronic monitor for metered dose inhalers. *Annals of Allergy, Asthma, & Immunology, 86*, 421–424.

Aronson, N., Lefevre, F., Piper, M., Mark, D., Bohn, R., Speroff, T., et al. (2001). *Management of chronic asthma.* Evidence Report/Technology Assessment Number 44. (Prepared by Blue

M.A. Rapoff, *Adherence to Pediatric Medical Regimens,* Issues in Clinical Child Psychology, DOI 10.1007/978-1-4419-0570-3,
© Springer Science+Business Media, LLC 2010

Cross and Blue Shield Association Technology Evaluation Center under Contract No. 290-97-0015). AHRQ Publication No. 01-E044. Rockville, MD: Agency for Healthcare Research and Quality. September 2001.

Averbuch, M., Weintraub, M., & Pollock, D. J. (1990). Compliance assessment in clinical trials. *Journal of Clinical Research and Pharmacoepidemiology, 4,* 199–204.

Backes, J. M., & Schentag, J. J. (1991). Partial compliance as a source of variance in pharmacokinetics and therapeutic drug monitoring. In J. A. C. B. Spilker (Ed.), *Patient compliance in medical practice and clinical trials* (pp. 27–36). New York: Raven Press.

Bandura, A. (1986). *Social foundations of thought and action: A social cognitive theory.* Englewood Cliffs, NJ: Prentice-Hall.

Bandura, A. (1995). Comments on the crusade against the causal efficacy of human thought. *Journal of Behavior Therapy and Experimental Psychiatry, 26,* 179–190.

Bandura, A. (1996). Ontological and epistemological terrains revisited. *Journal of Behavior Therapy & Experimental Psychiatry, 27,* 323–345.

Bandura, A. (1997). *Self-efficacy: The exercise of control.* New York: W.H. Freeman.

Barabino, A., Torrente, F., Ventura, A., Cucchiara, S., Castro, M., & Barbera, C. (2002). Azathioprine in paediatric inflammatory bowel disease: An Italian multicentre survey. *Alimentary Pharmacology & Therapeutics, 16,* 1125–1130.

Barakat, L. P., Smith-Whitley, K., & Ohene-Frempong, K. (2002). Treatment adherence in children with sickle cell disease: Disease-related risk and psychosocial factors. *Journal of Clinical Psychology in Medical Settings, 9,* 201–209.

Barlow, D. H., Nock, M. K., & Hersen, M. (2009). *Single case experimental designs: Strategies for studying behavior change* (3rd ed.) Boston: Pearson Education.

Barnard, M. U. (1986). Care of the child with type I diabetes. *Pediatric Nursing Update, 1,* 2–10.

Barrios, B. A. (1988). On the changing nature of behavioral assessment. In A. S. Bellack, & M. Hersen (Eds.), *Behavioral assessment: A practical handbook* (3rd ed., pp. 3–41). New York: Pergamon.

Bartholomew, L. K., Czyzewski, D. I., Parcel, G. S., Swank, P. R., Sockrider, M. M., Mariotto, M. J., et al. (1997). Self-management of cystic fibrosis: Short-term outcomes of the cystic fibrosis family education program. *Health Education & Behavior, 24,* 652–666.

Bartlett, S. J., Krishnan, J. A., Riekert, K. A., Butz, A. M., Malveaux, F. J., & Rand, C. S. (2004). Maternal depressive symptoms and adherence to therapy in inner-city children with asthma. *Pediatrics, 113,* 229–237.

Baum, D., & Creer, T. L. (1986). Medication compliance in children with asthma. *Journal of Asthma, 23,* 49–59.

Bauman, L. J., Drotar, D., Leventhal, J. M., Perrin, E. C., & Pless, I. B. (1997). A review of psychosocial interventions for children with chronic health conditions. *Pediatrics, 100,* 244–251.

Bauman, L. J., Wright, E., Leickly, F. E., Crain, E., Kruszon-Moran, D., Wade, S. L., et al. (2002). Relationship of adherence to pediatric asthma morbidity among inner-city children. *Pediatrics, 110,* 1–7.

Bazzigaluppi, E., Roggero, P., Parma, B., Brambillasca, M. F., Meroni, F., Mora, S., et al. (2006). Antibodies to recombinant human tissue-transglutaminase in coeliac disease: Diagnostic effectiveness and decline pattern after gluten-free diet. *Digestive and Liver Disease, 38,* 98–102.

Beck, D. E., Fennell, R. S., Yost, R. L., Robinson, J. D., Geary, D., & Richards, G. A. (1980). Evaluation of an educational program on compliance with medication regimens in pediatric patients with renal transplants. *The Journal of Pediatrics, 96,* 1094–1097.

Becker, M. H. (1974). The health belief model and personal health behavior. *Health Education Monographs, 2,* 324–508.

Bellack, A. S., & Hersen, M. (1988). *Behavioral assessment: A practical handbook* (3rd ed.). New York: Pergamon Press.

Bender, B., Milgrom, H., Rand, C., & Ackerson, L. (1998). Psychological factors associated with medication nonadherence in asthmatic children. *Journal of Asthma, 35*, 347–353.

Bender, B., Wamboldt, F. S., O'Connor, S. L., Rand, C., Szefler, S., Milgrom, H., et al. (2000). Measurement of children's asthma medication adherence by self report, mother report, canister weight, and Doser CT. *Annals of Allergy, Asthma, & Immunology, 85*, 416–421.

Bender, B. G., Pedan, A., & Varasteh, L. T. (2006). Adherence and persistence with fluticasone propionate/salmeterol combination therapy. *Journal of Allergy & Clinical Immunology, 118*, 899–904.

Benet, L. Z., Mitchell, J. R., & Sheiner, L. B. (1990). Pharmacokinetics: The dynamics of drug absorption, distribution, and elimination. In A. G. Gilman, T. W. Rall, A. S. Nies, & P. Taylor (Eds.), *Goodman and Gilman's: The pharmacological basis of therapeutics* (pp. 3–32). New York: Pergamon Press.

Berg, C. J., Rapoff, M. A., Snyder, C. R., & Belmont, J. M. (2007). The relationship of children's hope to pediatric asthma treatment adherence. *The Journal of Positive Psychology, 2*, 176–184.

Berg, J. S., Dischler, J., Wagner, D. J., Raia, J., & Palmer-Shevlin, N. (1993). Medication compliance: A health care problem. *The Annals of Pharmacotherapy, 27*(Suppl.), 2–21.

Bergman, A. B., & Werner, R. J. (1963). Failure of children to receive penicillin by mouth. *The New England Journal of Medicine, 268*, 1334–1338.

Berkovitch, M., Papadouris, D., Shaw, D., Onuoha, N., Dias, C., & Olivieri, N. F. (1998). Trying to improve compliance with prophylactic penicillin therapy in children with sickle cell disease. *British Journal of Clinical Pharmacology, 45*, 605–607.

Berrien, V. M., Salazar, J. C., Reynolds, E., & McKay, K. (2004). Adherence to antiretroviral therapy in HIV-infected pediatric patients improves with home-based intensive nursing intervention. *AIDS Patient Care and STDs, 18*, 355–363.

Bertakis, K. D. (1986). An application of the health belief model to patient education and compliance: Acute otitis media. *Family Medicine, 18*, 347–350.

Bloom, B. R., & Murray, C. J. L. (1992). Tuberculosis: Commentary on a reemergent killer. *Science, 257*, 1055–1064.

Blowey, D. L., Hebert, D., Arbus, G. S., Pool, R., Korus, M., & Koren, G. (1997). Compliance with cyclosporine in adolescent renal transplant recipients. *Pediatric Nephrology, 11*, 547–551.

Blue, J. W., & Colburn, W. A. (1996). Efficacy measures: Surrogates or clinical outcomes? *Journal of Clinical Pharmacology, 36*, 76–770.

Bobrow, E. S., AvRuskin, T. W., & Siller, J. (1985). Mother-daughter interaction and adherence to diabetes regimens. *Diabetes Care, 8*, 146–151.

Boccuti, L., Celano, M., Geller, R. J., & Phillips, K. M. (1996). Development of a scale to measure children's metered-dose inhaler and spacer technique. *Annals of Allergy, Asthma, & Immunology, 77*, 217–221.

Bond, G. G., Aiken, L. S., & Somerville, S. C. (1992). The health belief model and adolescents with insulin-dependent diabetes mellitus. *Health Psychology, 11*, 190–198.

Bond, W. S., & Hussar, D. A. (1991). Detection methods and strategies for improving medication compliance. *American Journal of Hospital Pharmacy, 48*, 1978–1988.

Bonner, S., Zimmerman, B. J., Evans, D., Irigoyen, M., Resnick, D., & Mellins, R. B. (2002). An individualized intervention to improve asthma management among urban Latino and African-American families. *Journal of Asthma, 39*, 167–179.

Boréus, L. O. (1989). The role of therapeutic drug monitoring in children. *Clinical Pharmacokinetics, 17*, 4–12.

Branstetter, A. D., Berg, C. J., Rapoff, M. A., & Belmont, J. M. (in press). Predicting children's adherence to asthma medication regimens. *Journal of Behavior Analysis in Sport, Health Fitness, and Medicine*.

Brewer, E. J., Giannini, E. H., Kuzmina, N., & Alekseev, L. (1986). Penicillamine and hydroxychloroquine in the treatment of severe juvenile rheumatoid arthritis. *The New England Journal of Medicine, 314*, 1269–1276.

Brooks-Gunn, J., & Graber, J. A. (1994). Puberty as a biological and social event: Implications for research on pharmacology. *Journal of Adolescent Health, 15*, 663–671.

Brown, S. J., Lieberman, D. A., Gemeny, B. A., Fan, Y. C., Wilson, D. M., & Pasta, D. J. (1997). Educational video game for juvenile diabetes: Results of a controlled trial. *Medical Informatics, 22*, 77–89.

Brownlee-Duffeck, M., Perterson, L., Simonds, J. F., Goldstein, D., Kilo, C., & Hoette, S. (1987). The role of health beliefs in the regimen adherence and metabolic control of adolescents and adults with diabetes mellitus. *Journal of Consulting and Clinical Psychology, 55*, 139–144.

Brownbridge, G., & Fielding, D. M. (1994). Psychosocial adjustment and adherence to dialysis treatment regimens. *Pediatric Nephrology, 8*, 744–749.

Brozekowski, D. L. G., Fobil, J. N., & Kofi, O. A. (2006). Online access by adolescents in Accra: Ghanaian teens' use of the internet for health information. *Developmental Psychology, 42*, 450–458.

Burkhart, P. V., Dunbar-Jacob, J. M., Fireman, P., & Rohay, J. (2002). Children's adherence to recommended asthma self-management. *Pediatric Nursing, 28*, 409–414.

Burkhart, P. V., Rayens, M. K., Oakley, M. G., Abshire, D. A., & Zhang, M. (2007). Testing an intervention to promote children's adherence to asthma self-management. *Journal of Nursing Scholarship, 39*, 133–140.

Burroughs, T. E., Pontious, S. L., & Santiago, J. V. (1993). The relationship among six psychosocial domains, age, health care adherence, and metabolic control in adolescents with IDDM. *Diabetes Education, 19*, 396–402.

Bursch, B., Schwankovsky, L., Gilbert, J., & Zeiger, R. (1999). Construction and validation of four childhood asthma self-management scales: Parent barriers, child and parent self-efficacy, and parent belief in treatment efficacy. *Journal of Asthma, 36*, 115–128.

Bush, P. J., & Iannotti, R. J. (1990). A children's health belief model. *Medical Care, 28*, 69–86.

Buston, K. M., & Wood, S. F. (2000). Non-compliance amongst adolescents with asthma: Listening to what they tell us about self-management. *Family Practice, 17*, 134–138.

Butz, A. M., Donithan, M., Bollinger, M. E., Rand, C., & Thompson, R. E. (2005). Monitoring nebulizer is in children: Comparison of electronic and asthma diary data. *Annals of Allergy Asthma and Immunology, 94*, 360–365.

Carney, R. M., Schechter, K., & Davis, T. (1983). Improving adherence to blood glucose testing in insulin-dependent diabetic children. *Behavior Therapy, 14*, 247–254.

Carton, J. S., & Schweitzer, J. B. (1996). Use of a token economy to increase compliance during hemodialysis. *Journal of Applied Behavior Analysis, 28*, 111–113.

Cary, J., Hein, K., & Dell, R. (1991). Theophylline disposition in adolescents with asthma. *Therapeutic Drug Monitoring, 13*, 309–313.

Casey, R., Rosen, B., Glowasky, A., & Ludwig, S. (1985). An intervention to improve follow-up of patients with otitis media. *Clinical Pediatrics, 24*, 149–152.

Cassell, E. J. (1991). *The nature of suffering and the goals of medicine.* New York: Oxford University Press.

Catania, A. C. (1995). Higher-order behavior classes: Contingencies, beliefs, and verbal behavior. *Journal of Behavior Therapy & Experimental Psychiatry, 26*, 191–200.

Celano, M., Geller, R. J., Phillips, K. M., & Ziman, R. (1998). Treatment adherence among low-income children with asthma. *Journal of Pediatric Psychology, 23*, 345–349.

Chan, D. S., Callahan, C. W., Hatch-Pigott, V. B., Lawless, A., Proffitt, H. L., Manning, N. E., et al. (2007). Internet-based home monitoring and education of children with asthma is comparable to ideal office-based care: Results of a 1-year asthma in-home monitoring trial. *Pediatrics, 119*, 569–578.

Charney, E., Bynum, R., Eldreye, D., Frank, D., MacWhinney, J. B., McNabb, N., et al. (1967). How well do patients take oral penicillin? A collaborative study in private practice. *Pediatrics, 40*, 188–195.

Chemlik, F., & Doughty, A. (1994). Objective measurement of compliance in asthma treatment. *Annals of Allergy, 73*, 527–532.

Cipani, E. (2004). *Punishment on trial*. Reno, NV: Context Press.

Clark, N. M., & Houle, C. R. (2009). Theoretical models and strategies for improving disease management by patients. In S. A. Shumaker, J. K. Ockene, & K. A. Riekert (Eds.), *The handbook of health behavior change* (3rd ed., pp. 19–37). New York: Springer.

Cleemput, I., Kesteloot, K., & DeGeest, S. (2002). A review of the literature on the economics of noncompliance. Room for methodological improvement. *Health Policy, 59*, 65–94.

Cluss, P. A., & Epstein, L. H. (1984). A riboflavin tracer method for assessment of medication compliance in children. *Behavior Research Methods, Instruments, & Computers, 16*, 444–446.

Cluss, P. A., Epstein, L. H., Galvis, S. A., Fireman, P., & Friday, G. (1984). Effect of compliance for chronic asthmatic children. *Journal of Consulting & Clinical Psychology, 52*, 909–910.

Cohen, J. (1988). *Statistical power analysis for the behavioral sciences* (2nd ed.). Hillsdale, NJ: Lawrence Erlbaum Associates.

Cohen, L. L., La Greca, A. M., Blount, R. L., Kazak, A. E., Holmbeck, G. N., & Lemanek, K. L. (2008a). Introduction to special issues: Evidence-based assessment in pediatric psychology. *Journal of Pediatric Psychology, 33*, 911–915.

Cohen, L. L., Lemanek, K., Blount, R. L., Dahlquist, L. M., Lim, C. S., Palermo, T. M., et al. (2008b). Evidence-based assessment of pediatric pain. *Journal of Pediatric Psychology, 33*, 939–955.

Colcher, I. S., & Bass, J. W. (1972). Penicillin treatment of streptococcal pharyngitis: A comparison of schedules and the role of specific counseling. *The Journal of the American Medical Association, 222*, 657–659.

Coleman, J. C., & Hendry, L. (1990). T*he nature of adolescence.* (2nd ed.). New York: Routledge.

Corcoran, K. J. (1995). Understanding cognition, choice, and behavior. *Journal of Behaviour Therapy & Experimental Psychiatry, 206*, 201–207.

Coutts, J. A. P., Gibson, N. A., & Paton, J. Y. (1992). Measuring compliance with inhaled medication in asthma. *Archives of Diseases of Children, 67*, 332–333.

Cramer, J. A. (1991). Overview of methods to measure and enhance patient compliance. In J. A. Cramer & B. Spilker (Eds.), *Patient compliance in medical practice and clinical trials* (pp. 3–10). New York: Raven Press.

Cramer, J. A. (1995). Microelectronic systems for monitoring and enhancing patient compliance with medication regimens. *Drugs, 49*, 321–327.

Crocker, L., & Algina, J. (1986). *Introduction to classical and modern test theory*. New York: Rinehart Winston.

Croft, D. R., & Peterson, M. W. (2002). An evaluation of the quality and contents of asthma education on the world wide web. *Chest, 121*, 1301–1307.

Cuffari, C., Théorêt, Y., & Seidman, L. (1996). 6-Mercaptopurine metabolism in Crohn's disease: Correlation with efficacy and toxicity. *Gut, 39*, 401–406.

Czajkowski, D. R., & Koocher, G. P. (1987). Medical compliance and coping with cystic fibrosis. *Journal of Child Psychology and Psychiatry, 28*, 311–319.

Czajkowski, S. M., Chesney, M. A., & Smith, A. W. (2009). Adherence and the placebo effect. In S. A. Shumaker, J. K. Ockene, & K. A. Riekert (Eds.), *The handbook of health behavior change* (3rd ed., pp. 713–734). New York: Springer.

da Costa, I. G., Rapoff, M. A., Lemanek, K., & Goldstein, G. L. (1997). Improving adherence to medication regimens for children with asthma and it's effect on clinical outcome. *Journal of Applied Behavior Analysis, 30*, 687–691.

Dahlström, B., & Eckernäs, S. A. (1991). Patient computers to enhance compliance with completing questionnaires: A challenge for the 1990's. In J. A. Cramer & B. Spilker (Eds.), *Patient compliance in medical practice and clinical trials* (pp. 233–240). New York: Raven Press.

Daschner, F., & Marget, W. (1975). Treatment of recurrent urinary tract infection in children. *Acta Paediatrica Scandivica, 54*, 105–108.

Davis, C. L., Delamater, A. M., Shaw, K. H., La Greca, A. M., Eidson, M. S., Perez-Rodriguez, J. E., et al. (2001). Parenting styles, regimen adherence, and glycemic control in 4- to 10-year-old children with diabetes. *Journal of Pediatric Psychology, 26*, 123–129.

Davis, M. A., Quittner, A. L., Stack, C. M., & Yang, M. C. K. (2004). Controlled evaluation of the STARBRIGHT CD-ROM program for children and adolescents with cystic fibrosis. *Journal of Pediatric Psychology, 29*, 259–267.

Dawes, R. M., Faust, D., & Meehl, P. E. (1989). Clinical versus actuarial judgment. *Science, 243*, 1668–1674.

Dawson, K. P., & Jamieson, A. (1971). Value of blood phenytoin estimation in management of childhood epilepsy. *Archives of Disease in Childhood, 46*, 386–388.

Deaton, A. V. (1985). Adaptive noncompliance in pediatric asthma: The parent as expert. *Journal of Pediatric Psychology, 10*, 1–14.

Deci, E. L., & Ryan, R. M. (1985). *Intrinsic motivation and self-determination in human behavior.* New York: Plenum.

Delamater, A. M., Applegate, B., Shaw, K. H., Edison, M., Szapocznik, J., & Nemery, R. (1997). What accounts for poor metabolic control in minority youths with diabetes? *Annals of Behavioral Medicine, 19* (Suppl.), S064.

DeLambo, K. E., Ievers-Landis, C. E., Drotar, D., & Quittner, A. L. (2004). Association of observed family relationship quality and problem-solving skills with treatment adherence in older children and adolescents with cystic fibrosis. *Journal of Pediatric Psychology, 29*, 343–353.

Demir, H., Yüce, A., Caglar, M., Kale, G., Kocak, N., Özen, H., et al. (2005). Cirrhosis in children with celiac disease. *Journal of Clinical Gastroenterology, 39*, 630–633.

Denson-Lino, J. M., Willies-Jacobo, L. J., Rosas, A., O'Connor, R. D., & Wilson, N. W. (1993). Effect of economic status on the use of house dust mite avoidance measures in asthmatic children. *Annals of Allergy, 71*, 130–132.

DeVellis, B. M., & DeVellis, R. F. (2001). Self-efficacy and health. In A. Baum, T. A. Revenson, & J. E. Singer (Eds.), *Handbook of health psychology* (pp. 235–247). Mahwah, NJ: Lawrence Erlbaum Associates.

Devries, J. M., & Hoekelman, R. A. (1988). Comparison of four methods of assessing compliance with a medication regimen: Parent interview, medication diary, unused medication measurement, and urinary drug excretion. *American Journal of Diseases in Children, 142*, 396.

Dickey, F. F., Mattar, M. E., & Chudziker, G. M. (1975). Pharmacist counseling increases drug regimen compliance. *Hospitals, 49*, 85–89.

DiClemente, C., Prochaska, J. O., Fairhurst, S. R., Velicer, W. F., Velasquez, M. M., & Rossi, J. S. (1991). The process of smoking cessation: An analysis of precontemplation, contemplation, and preparation stages of change. *Journal of Consulting & Clinical Psychology, 59*, 295–304.

DiClemente, C. C., & Prochaska, J. O. (1982). Self-change and therapy change of smoking behavior: A comparison of process of change in cessation and maintenance. *Addictive Behaviors, 7*, 133–142.

DiMatteo, M. R., & DiNicola, D. D. (1982). *Achieving patient compliance: The psychology of the medical practitioner's role.* New York: Pergamon.

Disney, F. A., Francis, A. B., Breese, B. B., Green, J. L., & Talpey, W. B. (1979). The use of cefaclor in the treatment of beta-haemolytic streptococcal throat infections in children. *Postgraduate Medical Journal, 55*, 50–52.

Dohil, R., Hassall, E., Wadsworth, L. D., & Israel, D. M. (1998). Recombinant human erythropoietin for treatment of anemia of chronic disease in children with Crohn's disease. *The Journal of Pediatrics, 132*, 155–159.

Dolezal, C., Mellins, C., Brackis-Cott, E., & Abrams, E. J. (2003). The reliability of reports of medical adherence from children with HIV and their adult caregivers. *Journal of Pediatric Psychology, 28*, 355–361.

Downs, J. A., Roberts, C. M., Blackmore, A. M., Le Souëf, P. N., & Jenkins, S. C. (2006). Benefits of an education programme on the self-management of aerosol and airway clearance treatments for children with cystic fibrosis. *Chronic Respiratory Disease, 3*, 19–27.

Dracup, K. A., & Meleis, A. I. (1982). Compliance: An interactionist approach. *Nursing Research, 31*, 31–36.

Drotar, D., Greenley, R., Hoff, A., Johnson, C., Lewandowski, A., Moore, M., et al. (2006). Summary of issues and challenges in the use of new technologies in clinical care and with children and adolescents with chronic illness. *Children's Health Care, 35*, 91–102.

Dunbar, J. M., Marshall, G. D., & Hovell. (1979). Behavioral strategies for improving compliance. In R. B. Haynes, D. W. Taylor, & D. L. Sackett (Eds.), *Compliance in health care* (pp. 174–190). Baltimore: The Johns Hopkins University Press.

Eggleston, P. A., Malveaux, F. J., Butz, A. M., Huss, K., Thompson, L., Kolodner, K., et al., (1998). Medications used by children with asthma living in the inner city. *Pediatrics, 101*, 349–354.

Eisenberger, R., & Cameron, J. (1996). Detrimental effects of reward: Reality or myth? *American Psychologist, 51*, 1153–1166.

Eiser, C., & Morse, R. (2001). The measurement of quality of life in children: Past and future perspectives. *Journal of Developmental & Behavioral Pediatrics, 22*, 248–256.

El-Charr, G. M., Mardy, G., Wehlou, K., & Rubin, L. G. (1996). Randomized, double blind comparison of brand and generic antibiotic suspensions: II. A study of taste and compliance in children. *Pediatric Infectious Diseases Journal, 15*, 18–22.

Ellis, D. A., Frey, M. A., Naar-King, S., Templin, T., Cunningham, P., & Cakan, N. (2005). Use of multisystemic therapy to improve regimen adherence among adolescents with type 1 diabetes in chronic poor metabolic control: A randomized controlled trial. *Diabetes Care, 28*, 1604–1610.

Ellis, D. A., Naar-King, S., Cunningham, P. B., & Secord, E. (2006). Use of multisystemic therapy to improve antiretroviral adherence and health outcomes in HIV-infected pediatric patients: Evaluation of a pilot program. *AIDS Patient Care and STDs, 20*, 112–121.

Ellis, D. A., Podolski, C., Frey, M., Naar-King, S., Wang, B., & Moltz, K. (2007). The role of parental monitoring in adolescent health outcomes: Impact of regimen adherence in youth with type 1 diabetes. *Journal of Pediatric Psychology, 32*, 907–917.

Ellis, D. A., Templin, T. N., Naar-King, S., & Frey, M. (2008). Toward conceptual clarity in a critical parenting construct: Parental monitoring in youth with chronic illness. *Journal of Pediatric Psychology, 33*, 799–808.

Ellis, D. A., Yopp, J., Templin, T., Naar-King, S., Frey, M. A., Cunningham, P. B., et al. (2007). Family mediators and moderators of treatment outcomes among youths with poorly controlled type 1 diabetes: Results from a randomized controlled trial. *Journal of Pediatric Psychology, 32*, 194–205.

Ellison, R. S., & Altemeier, W. A. (1982). Effect of use of a measured dispensing device on oral antibiotic compliance. *Clinical Pediatrics, 21*, 668–671.

Eney, R. D., & Goldstein, E. O. (1976). Compliance of chronic asthmatics with oral administration of theophylline as measured by serum and salivary levels. *Pediatrics, 57*, 513–517.

Epstein, L. H. (1984). The direct effects of compliance on health outcome. *Health Psychology, 3*, 385–393.

Epstein, L. H., Figueroa, J., Farkas, G. M., & Beck, S. (1981). The short-term effects of feedback on accuracy of urine glucose determinations in insulin dependent diabetic children. *Behavior Therapy, 12*, 560–564.

Ertekin, V., Selimoğlu, A., Türkan, Y., & Akçay, F. (2005). Serum nitric oxide levels in children with celiac disease. *Journal of Clinical Gastroenterology, 39*, 782–785.

Ettenger, R. B., Rosenthal, J. T., Marik, J. L., Malekzadeh, M., Forsythe, S. B., Kamil, E. S., et al. (1991). Improved cadaveric renal transplant outcome in children. *Pediatric Nephrology, 5*, 137–142.

Farley, J., Hines, S., Musk, A., Ferrus, S., & Tepper, V. (2003). Assessment of adherence to antiviral therapy in HIV-infected children using the medication event monitoring system, pharmacy refill, provider assessment, caregiver self-report, and appointment keeping. *Journal of Acquired Immune Deficiency Syndromes, 33*, 211–218.

Farmer, K. C. (1999). Methods for measuring and monitoring medication regimen adherence in clinical trials and clinical practice. *Clinical Therapeutics, 21*, 1074–1090.

Feinstein, S., Keich, R., Becker-Cohen, R., Rinat, C., Schwartz, S. B., & Frishberg, Y. (2005). Is noncompliance among adolescent renal transplant recipients inevitable? *Pediatrics, 115*, 969–973.

Feldman, D. E., De Civita, M., Dobkin, P. L., Malleson, P., Meshefedjian, G., & Duffy, C. (2007). Perceived adherence to prescribed treatment in juvenile idiopathic arthritis over a one-year period. *Arthritis Care & Research, 57*, 226–233.

Feldman, W., Momy, J., & Dulberg, C. (1988). Trimethoprin-sulfamethoxazole vs. amoxicillin in the treatment of acute otitis media. *Canadian Medical Association Journal, 139*, 961–964.

Fennell, R. S., Foulkes, L. M., & Boggs, S. R. (1994). Family-based program to promote medication compliance in renal transplant children. *Transplantation Proceedings, 26*, 102–103.

Festa, R. S., Tamaroff, M. H., Chasalow, F., & Lanzkowsky, P. (1992). Therapeutic adherence to oral medication regimens by adolescents with cancer. I. Laboratory assessment. *Journal of Pediatrics, 120*, 807–811.

Fink, D., Malloy, M. J., Cohen, M., Greycloud, M. A., & Martin, F. (1969). Effective patient care in the pediatric ambulatory setting: A study of the acute care clinic. *Pediatrics, 43*, 927–935.

Finney, J. W., Friman, P. C., Rapoff, M. A., & Christophersen, E. R. (1985). Improving compliance with antibiotic regimens for otitis media: Randomized clinical trial in a pediatric clinic. *American Journal of Diseases in Children, 139*, 89–95.

Finney, J. W., Hook, R. J., Friman, P. C., Rapoff, M. A., & Christophersen, E. R. (1993). The overestimation of adherence to pediatric medical regimens. *Children's Health Care, 22*, 297–304.

Fishbein, M. (1967). *Readings in attitude theory and measurement*. New York: Wiley.

Fisher, C. B., & Fried, A. L. (2003). Internet-mediated psychological services and the American Psychological Association ethics code. *Psychotherapy: Theory, Research, Practice, Training, 40*, 103–111.

Fletcher, R. H., Fletcher, S. W., & Wagner, E. H. (1988). *Clinical epidemiology: The essentials*. (2nd ed.). Baltimore: Williams & Wilkins.

Forbis, S., & Aligne, C. A. (2002). Poor readability of written asthma management plans found in national guidelines. *Pediatrics, 109*, e52.

Foster, S. L., Bell-Dolan, D. J., & Burge, D. A. (1988). Behavioral observation. In A. S. Bellack & M. Hersen (Eds.), *Behavioral assessment: A practical handbook* (3rd ed., pp. 119–160). New York: Pergamon Press.

Fredericks, E. M., Magee, J. C., Opipari-Arrigan, L., Shieck, V., Well, A., & Lopez, M. J. (2008). Adherence and health-related quality of life in adolescent liver transplant recipients. *Pediatric Transplantation, 12*, 289–299.

Freund, A., Johnson, S. B., Silverstein, J., & Thomas, J. (1991). Assessing daily management of childhood diabetes using the 24-hour recall interviews: Reliability and stability. *Health Psychology, 10*, 200–208.

Friedman, I. M., Litt, I. F., King, D. R., Henson, R., Holtzman, D., Halverson, D., et al. (1986). Compliance with anticonvulsant therapy by epileptic youth. *Journal of Adolescent Health Care, 7*, 12–17.

Friman, P. C. (2009). Behavior assessment. In D. H. Barlow, M. K. Nock, & M. Hersen (Eds.), *Single case experimental designs: Strategies for studying behavior change* (3rd ed., pp. 99–134). Boston: Pearson Education.

Garvie, P. A., Lensing, S., & Rai, S. N. (2007). Efficacy of a pill-swallowing training intervention to improve antiretroviral medication adherence in pediatric patients with HIV/AIDS. *Pediatrics, 119*, e893–e899.

Geiss, S. K., Hobbs, S. A., Hammersley-Maercklein, G., Kramer, J. C., & Henley, M. (1992). Psychosocial factors related to perceived compliance with cystic fibrosis treatment. *Journal of Clinical Psychology, 48*, 99–103.

Gelfand, K., Geffken, G., Halsey-Lyda, M., Muir, A., & Malasanos, T. (2003). Intensive telehealth management of five at-risk adolescents with diabetes. *Journal of Telemedicine and Telecare, 9*, 117–121.

Gerber, M. A., Randolph, M. F., Chanatry, J., Wright, L. L., Anderson, L. R., & Kaplan, E. L. (1986). Once daily therapy for streptococcal pharyngitis with cefadroxil. *Journal of Pediatrics, 109*, 531–537.

Gerson, A. C., Furth, S. L., Neu, A. M., & Fivush, B. A. (2004). Assessing associations between medication adherence and potentially modifiable psychosocial variables in pediatric kidney transplant recipients and their families. *Pediatric Transplantation, 8*, 543–550.

Giannini, E. H. Brewer, E. J., Miller, M. L., Gibbas, D., Passo, M. H., Hoyeraal, H. M., et al. (1990). Ibuprofen suspension in the treatment of juvenile rheumatoid arthritis. *Journal of Pediatrics, 117*, 645–652.

Gibbons, A. (1992). Exploring new strategies to fight drug-resistant microbes. *Science, 257*, 1036–1038.

Gilbert, A., & Varni, J. W. (1988). Behavioral treatment for improving adherence to factor replacement therapy by children with hemophilia. *The Journal of Compliance in Health Care, 3*, 67–76.

Gilbert, B. O., Johnson, S. B., Spillar, R., McCallum, M., Silverstein, J. H., & Rosenbloom, A. (1982). The effects of a peer-modeling film on children learning to self-inject insulin. *Behavior Therapy, 13*, 186–193.

Gilbert, D. T., & Malone, P. S. (1995). The correspondence bias. *Psychological Bulletin, 117*, 21–38.

Gibson, N. A., Ferguson, A. E., Aitchison, T. C., & Paton, J. Y. (1995). Compliance with inhaled asthma medication in preschool children. *Thorax, 50*, 1274–1279.

Gill, T. M., & Feinstein, A. R. (1994). A critical appraisal of the quality of quality-of-life measurements. *Journal of the America Medical Association, 272*, 619–626.

Ginsburg, C. M., McCracken, G. H., Steinberg, J. B., Crow, S. D., Dildy, B. F., Cope, F., et al. (1982). Treatment of group A streptococcal pharyngitis in children: Results of a prospective, randomized study of four antimicrobial agents. *Clinical Pediatrics, 21*, 83–88.

Glasgow, R. E., McCaul, K. D., & Schafer, L. C. (1986). Barriers to regimen adherence among persons with insulin-dependent diabetes. *Journal of Behavioral Medicine, 9*, 65–77.

Goldring, J. M., James, D. S., & Anderson, H. A. (1993). Chronic lung diseases. In P. L. Brownson & J. R. Davis (Eds.), *Chronic disease epidemiology and control* (pp. 169–197). Washington, DC: American Public Health Association.

Goldstein, A., & Sculerati, N. (1994). Compliance with prophylactic antibiotics for otitis media in a New York City clinic. *International Journal of Pediatric Otorhinolaryngology, 28*, 129–140.

Goodwin, D. A. J., Boggs, S. R., & Graham-Pole, J. (1994). Development and validation of the pediatric oncology quality of life scale. *Psychological Assessment, 6*, 321–328.

Gordis, L. (1979). Conceptual and methodologic problems in measuring patient compliance. In R. B. Haynes, D. W. Taylor, & D. L. Sackett (Eds.), *Compliance in health care* (pp. 23–45). Baltimore: The Johns Hopkins University Press.

Gordis, L., & Markowitz, M. (1971). Evaluation of the effectiveness of comprehensive and continuous pediatric care. *Pediatrics, 48*, 766–776.

Gordis, L., Markowitz, M., & Lilienfeld, A. M. (1969). The inaccuracy in using interviews to estimate patient reliability in taking medications at home. *Medical Care, 7*, 49–54.

Graves, M. M., Roberts, M. C., Rapoff, M. A., & Boyer, A. (in press). The efficacy of adherence interventions for chronically ill children: A meta-analytic review. *Journal of Pediatric Psychology.*

Gray, N. J., Klein, J. D., Noyce, P. R., Sesselberg, T. S., & Cantrill, J. A. (2005). Health information-seeking behaviour in adolescence: The place of the internet. *Social Science & Medicine, 60*, 1467–1478.

Greco, P., La Greca, A. M., Ireland, S., Wick, P., Freeman, C., Agramonte, R., et al. (1990). Assessing adherence in IDDM: A comparison of two methods. *Diabetes Care, 40*(Suppl. 2), 108A, 165.

Greenan-Fowler, E., Powell, C., & Varni, J. W. (1987). Behavioral treatment of adherence to therapeutic exercise by children with hemophilia. *Archives of Physical Medicine & Rehabilitation, 68*, 846–849.

Greening, L., Stoppelbein, L., Konishi, C., Jordan, S. S., & Moll, G. (2007). Child routines and youths' adherence to treatment for type 1 diabetes. *Journal of Pediatric Psychology, 32,* 437–447.

Groopman, J. (2007). *How doctors think.* New York: Houghton Mifflin.

Gross, A. M. (1983). Self-management training and medication compliance in children with diabetes. *Child & Family Behavior Therapy, 4,* 47–55.

Gross, A. M., Magalnick, L. J., & Richardson, P. (1985). Self-management training with families of insulin-dependent diabetic children: A controlled long-term investigation. *Child & Family Behavior Therapy, 7,* 35–50.

Grossman, H. Y., Brink, S., & Hauser, S. T. (1987). Self-efficacy in adolescent girls and boys with insulin-dependent diabetes mellitus. *Diabetes Care, 10,* 324–329.

Gudas, L. J., Koocher, G. P., & Wyplj, D. (1991). Perceptions of medical compliance in children and adolescents with cystic fibrosis. *Developmental & Behavioral Pediatrics, 12,* 236–247.

Guerin, B. (1994). *Analyzing social behavior: Behavior analysis and the social sciences.* Reno, NV: Context Press.

Guevara, J. P., Wolf, F. M., Grum, C. M., & Clark, N. M. (2003). Effects of educational interventions for self management of asthma in children and adolescents: Systematic review and meta-analysis. *British Medical Journal, 326,* 1–6.

Hagopian, L. P., & Thompson, R. H. (1999). Reinforcement of compliance with respiratory treatment in a child with cystic fibrosis. *Journal of Applied Behavior Analysis, 32,* 233–236.

Halterman, J. S., Yoos, L., Kaczorowski, J. M., McConnochie, K., Holzhauer, R. J., Conn, K. M., et al. (2002). Providers underestimate symptom severity among urban children with asthma. *Archives of Pediatrics & Adolescent Medicine, 156,* 141–146.

Hanson, C. L., Cigrang, J. A., Harris, M. A., Carle, D. L., Relyea, G., & Burghen, G. A. (1989). Coping styles in youths with insulin-dependent diabetes mellitus. *Journal of Consulting and Clinical Psychology, 57,* 644–651.

Hanson, C. L., DeGuire, M. J., Schinkel, A. M., Kolterman, O. G., Goodman, J. P., & Buckingham, B. A. (1996). Self-care behaviors in insulin-dependent diabetes: Evaluative tools and their associations with glycemic control. *Journal of Pediatric Psychology, 21,* 467–482.

Hanson, C. L., Henggler, S. W., Harris, M. A., Cigrang, J. A., Schinkel, A. M., Rodrigue, J. R., et al. (1992). Contributions of sibling relations to the adaptation of youths with insulin-dependent diabetes mellitus. *Journal of Consulting and Clinical Psychology, 60,* 104–112.

Hartman, C., Hino, B., Lerner, A., Eshach-Adiv, O., Berkowitz, D., Shaoul, R., et al. (2004). Bone quantitative ultrasound and bone mineral density in children with celiac disease. *Journal of Pediatric Gastroenterology and Nutrition, 39,* 504–510.

Haskard, K. B., DiMatteo, M. R., & Williams, S. L. (2009). Adherence and health outcomes: How much does adherence matter? In S. A. Shumaker, J. K. Ockene, & K. A. Riekert (Eds.), *The handbook of health behavior change* (3rd ed., pp. 771–784). New York: Springer.

Hauser, S. T., Jacobson, A. M., Lavori, P., Wolfsdorf, J. I., Herskowite, R. D., Milley, J. E., & Bloss, R. (1990). Adherence among children and adolescents with insulin-dependent diabetes mellitus over a four-year longitudinal follow-up: II. Immediate and long-term linkages with the family milieu. *Journal of Pediatric Psychology, 15,* 527–542.

Hawkins, R. M. F. (1992). Self-efficacy: A predictor but not a cause of behavior. *Journal of Behavior Therapy & Experimental Psychiatry, 23,* 251–256.

Hawkins, R. M. F. (1995). Self-efficacy: A cause of debate. *Journal of Behavior Therapy & Experimental Psychiatry, 26,* 235–240.

Hayes, S. C. (Ed.). (1989). *Rule-governed behavior: Cognition, contingencies, and instructional control.* New York: Plenum.

Hayes, S. C., Kohlenberg, B. S., & Melancon, S. M. (1989). Avoiding and altering rule-control as a strategy of clinical intervention. In S. C. Hayes (Ed.), *Rule-governed behavior: Cognition, contingencies, and instructional control* (pp. 359–385). New York: Plenum.

Hayes, S. C., Nelson, R. O., & Jarrett, R. B. (1987). The treatment utility of assessment: A functional approach to evaluation assessment quality. *American Psychologist, 42,* 963–974.

Hayes, S. C., Strosahl, K. D., & Wilson, K. G. (1999). *Acceptance and commitment therapy: An experiential approach to behavior change*. New York: Guildford Press.

Hayes, S. C., & Wilson, K. G. (1995). The role of cognition in complex human behavior: A contextualistic perspective. *Journal of Behaviour Therapy & Experimental Psychiatry, 26*, 241–248.

Hayford, J. R., & Ross, C. K. (1988). Medical compliance in juvenile rheumatoid arthritis: Problems and perspectives. *Arthritis Care and Research, 1*, 190–197.

Haynes, R. B. (1979). Introduction. In D. W. Taylor & D. C. Sackett (Eds.), *Compliance in health care* (pp. 1–7). Baltimore: The Johns Hopkins University Press.

Haynes, R. B., Ackloo, E., Sahota, N., McDonald, H. P., & Yao, X. (2008). Interventions for enhancing medical adherence. *Cochrane Database of Systemic Reviews*, Issue 2. Art.No.: CD000011. DOI: 10.1002/14651858.CD000011.pub3.

Haynes, R. B., McKibbon, K. A., & Kanani, R. (1996). Systematic review of randomized trials of interventions to assist patients to follow prescriptions for medications. *Lancet, 348*, 383–386.

Haynes, R. B., Taylor, D. W., & Sackett, D. L. (1979). *Compliance in health care*. Baltimore: The Johns Hopkins University Press.

Haynes, S. M. (1992). *Models of causality in psychopathology*. New York: Macmillan.

Haynes, S. N., & O'Brien, W. H. (1990). Functional analysis in behavior therapy. *Clinical Psychology Review, 10*, 649–668.

Hazzard, A., Hutchinson, S. J., & Krawiecki, N. (1990). Factors related to adherence to medication regimens in pediatric seizure patients. *Journal of Pediatric Psychology, 15*, 543–555.

Heath, K. V., Singer, J., O'Shaughnessy, M. V., Montaner, J. S. G., & Hogg, R. S. (2002). Intentional nonadherence due to adverse symptoms associated with antiretroviral therapy. *Journal of Acquired Immune Deficiency Syndromes, 31*, 211–217.

Heidgerken, A. D., Adkins, J., Storch, E. A., Williams, L., Lewin, A. B., Silverstein, J. H., et al., (2006). Telehealth intervention for adolescents with type 1 diabetes. *The Journal of Pediatrics, 148*, 707–708.

Heisenberg, W. (1958). *Physics and philosophy: The revolution in modern science*. New York: Harper and Row.

Henness, D. M. (1982). A clinical experience with cefadroxil in upper respiratory tract infection. *Journal of Antimicrobial Chemotherapy, 10*, 125–135.

Hentinen, M., & Kyngas, H. (1992). Compliance of young diabetics with health regimens. *Journal of Advanced Nursing, 17*, 530–536.

Hobbs, S. A., Schweitzer, J. B., Cohen, L. L., Hayes, A. L., Schoell, C., & Crain, B. K. (2003). Maternal attributions related to compliance with cystic fibrosis treatment. *Journal of Clinical Psychology in Medical Settings, 10*, 273–277.

Holmbeck, G. N., Belvedere, M. C., Christensen, M., Czerwinski, A. M., Hommeyer, J. S., Johnson, S. Z., et al. (1998). Assessment of adherence with multiple informants in pre-adolescents with spina bifida: Initial development of a multidimensional, multitask parent-report questionnaire. *Journal of Personality Assessment, 70*, 427–440.

Holmes, C. S., Chen. R., Streisand, R., Marschall, D. E., Souter, S., Swift, E. E., et al. (2006). Predictors of youth diabetes care behaviors and metabolic control: A structural equation modeling approach. *Journal of Pediatric Psychology, 31*, 770–784.

Hommel, K. A., Davis, C. M., & Baldassano, R. N. (2008). Medication adherence and quality of life in pediatric inflammatory bowel disease. *Journal of Pediatric Psychology, 33*, 867–874.

Hoppe, J. E., Blumenstock, G., Grotz, W., Med, C., & Selbmann, H. (1999). Compliance of German pediatric patients with oral antibiotic therapy: Results of a nationwide survey. *The Pediatric Infectious Disease Journal, 18*, 1085–1091

Horner, R. H. (1994). Functional assessment: Contributions and future directions. *Journal of Applied Behavior Analysis, 27*, 401–404.

Horwitz, R. I., & Horwitz, S. M. (1993). Adherence to treatment and health outcomes. *Archives of Internal Medicine, 153*, 1863–1868.

Howe, C. J., Jawad, A. F., Tuttle, A. K., Moser, J. T., Preis, C. Buzby, M. et al. (2005). Education and telephone case management for children with type 1 diabetes: A randomized controlled trial. *Journal of Pediatric Nursing, 20*, 83–95.

Howe, S., Levinson, J., Shear, E., Hartner, S., McGirr, G., Schulte, M., et al. (1991). Development of a disability measurement tool for juvenile rheumatoid arthritis: The juvenile arthritis functional assessment report for children and their parents. *Arthritis & Rheumatism, 34*, 873–880.

Iannotti, R. J., Schneider, S., Nansel, T. R., Haynie, D. L., Plotnick, L. P., Clark, L. M., et al. (2006). Self-efficacy, outcome expectations, and diabetes self-management in adolescents with type 1 diabetes. *Journal of Developmental and Behavioral Pediatrics, 27*, 98–105.

Ingersoll, G. M., Orr, D. P. Herrold, A. J., & Golden, M. P. (1986). Cognitive maturity and self-management among adolescents with insulin-dependent diabetes mellitus. *Journal of Pediatrics, 108*, 620–623.

Insull, W. (1984). Statement of the problem and pharmacological and clinical requirements for the ideal marker. *Controlled Clinical Trials.* Dec;5(Suppl. 4), 459–462.

Ievers, C. E., Drotar, D., Dahms, W. T., Doershuk, C. F., & Stern, R. S. (1994). Maternal child-rearing behavior in three groups: Cystic fibrosis, insulin-dependent diabetes mellitus and healthy children. *Journal of Pediatric Psychology, 19*, 681–687.

Jacobson, A. M., Hauser, S. T., Lavori, P., Wolfsdorf, J. I., Herskowitz, R. D., Milley, J. E., et al. (1990). Adherence among children and adolescents with insulin-dependent diabetes mellitus over a four year longitudinal follow-up: I. The influence of patient coping and adjustment. *Journal of Pediatric Psychology, 15*, 511–526.

Jacobson, A. M., Hauser, S. T., Wolfsdorf, J. I., Houlihan, J., Milley, J. E., Hrskowitz, R. et al., (1987). Psychologic predictors of compliance in children with recent onset diabetes mellitus. *Journal of Pediatrics, 110*, 805–811.

Janz, N. K., & Becker, M. H. (1984). The health belief model: A decade later. *Health Education Quarterly, 11*, 1–47.

Jarzembowski, T., John, E., Panaro, F., Heiliczer, J., Kraft, K., Bogetti, D., et al., (2004). Impact of non-compliance on outcome after pediatric kidney transplantation: An analysis in racial subgroups. *Pediatric Transplantation, 8*, 367–371.

Jensen, S. A., Elkin, T. D., Hilker, K., Jordan, S., Iyer, R., & Smith, M. G. (2005). Caregiver knowledge and adherence in children with sickle cell disease: Knowing is not doing. *Journal of Clinical Psychology in Medical Settings, 12*, 333–337.

Johanson, C. E. (1992). Biochemical mechanisms and pharmacological principles of drug action. In J. Grabowski & G. R. Vandenbos (Eds.), *Psychopharmacology: Basic mechanisms and applied interventions* (pp. 15–58). Washington, DC: American Psychological Association.

Johnson, S. B. (1993). Chronic diseases of childhood: Assessing compliance with complex medical regimens. In M. A. Krasnegor, L. Epstein, S. B. Johnson, & S. J. Yaffe (Eds.), *Developmental aspects of health compliance behavior* (pp. 15–184). Hillsdale, NJ: Lawrence Erlbaum.

Johnson, S. B. (1994). Health behavior and health status: Concepts, methods and applications. *Journal of Pediatric Psychology, 19*, 129–141.

Johnson, S. B. (1995). Managing insulin-dependent diabetes mellitus in adolescence: A developmental perspective. In J. L. Wallander & L. J. Siegel (Eds.), *Adolescent health problems: Behavioral perspectives* (pp. 265–288). New York: Guilford.

Johnson, S. B., Freund, A., Silverstein, J., Hansen, C. A., & Malone, J. (1990). Adherence-health status relationships in childhood diabetes. *Health Psychology, 9*, 606–631.

Johnson, S. B., Kelly, M., Henretta, J. C., Cunningham, W. R., Tomer, A., & Silverstein, J. H. (1992). A longitudinal analysis of adherence and health status in childhood diabetes. *Journal of Pediatric Psychology, 17*, 537–553.

Johnston, J. M., & Pennypacker, H. S. (1993). *Strategies and tactics of behavioral research.* (2nd ed.). Hillsdale, NJ: Lawrence Erlbaum.

Jónasson, G., Carlsen, K.-H., & Mowinckel, P. (2000). Asthma drug adherence in a long term clinical trial. *Archives of Disease in Childhood, 83*, 330–333.

Julius, S. M., Sherman, J. M., & Hendeles, L. (2002). Accuracy of three electronic monitors for metered-dose inhalers. *Chest, 121*, 871–876.

Juniper, E. F., Guyatt, G. H., Feeny, D. H., Ferrie, P. J., Griffith, L. E., & Townsend, M. (1996). Measuring quality of life in children with asthma. *Quality of Life Research, 5*, 35–46.

Kahana, S., Drotar, D., & Frazier, T. (2008). Meta-analysis of psychological interventions to promote adherence to treatment in pediatric chronic health conditions. *Journal of Pediatric Psychology, 33*, 590–611.

Kamps, J. L., Rapoff, M. A., Roberts, M. C., Varela, R. E., Barnard, M., & Olson, N. (2008). Improving adherence to inhaled corticosteroids in children with asthma: A pilot of a randomized clinical trial. *Children's Health Care, 37*, 261–277.

Kaplan, R. M. (1994). The Ziggy theorem: Toward an outcomes-focused health psychology. *Health Psychology, 13*, 451–460.

Kaplan, R. M., & Simon, H. J. (1990). Compliance in medical care: Reconsiderations of self-predictions. *Annals of Behavioral Medicine, 12*, 66–71.

Kastrissios, H., Flowers, N. T., & Blaschke, T. F. (1996). Introducing medical students to medication noncompliance. *Clinical Pharmacology & Therapeutics, 59*, 577–582.

Kazak, A. E. (1997). A contextual family/systems approach to pediatric psychology: Introduction to the special issue. *Journal of Pediatric Psychology, 22*, 141–148.

Kazdin, A. E. (1977). Artifact, bias, and complexity of assessment: The ABCs of reliability. *Journal of Applied Behavior Analysis, 10*, 141–150.

Kazdin, A. E. (1994). *Behavior modification in applied settings* (5th ed.). Pacific Grove, CA: Brooks/Cole.

Kazdin, A. E. (2000). *Behavior modification in applied settings* (6th ed.). Florence, KY: Wadsworth/Cengage Learning.

Kelloway, J. S., Wyatt, R. A., & Adlis, S. A. (1994). Comparison of patients' compliance with prescribed oral and inhaled asthma medications. *Archives of Internal Medicine, 154*, 1349–1352.

Kendall, P. C. (1993). Cognitive-behavioral therapies with youth: Guiding theory, current status, and emerging developments. *Journal of Consulting and Clinical Psychology, 61*, 235–247.

Kennard, B. D., Stewart, S. M., Olvera, R., Bawdon, R. E., O Ailin, A., Lewis, C. P., et al. (2004). Nonadherence in adolescent oncology patients: Preliminary data on psychological risk factors and relationship to outcome. *Journal of Clinical Psychology in Medical Settings, 11*, 31–39.

Klinnert, M. D., McQuaid, E. L., & Gavin, L. A. (1997). Assessing the family asthma management system. *Journal of Asthma, 34*, 77–88.

Kolaček, S., Jadrešin, O., Petković, I., Mišak, Z., Sonicki, Z., & Booth, I. W. (2004). Gluten-free diet has a beneficial effect on chromosome instability in lymphocytes of children with coeliac disease. *Journal of Pediatric Gastroenterology and Nutrition, 38*, 177–180.

Kovacs, M., Goldsten, D., Obrosky, D. S., & Iyengar, S. (1992). Prevalence and predictors of pervasive noncompliance with medical treatment among youths with insulin-dependent diabetes mellitus. *Journal of the American Academy of Child and Adolescent Psychiatry, 31*, 1112–1119.

Kratochwill, T. R. (1985). Selection of target behaviors: Issues and directions. *Behavioral Assessment, 7*, 3–5.

Krishna, S., Francisco, B. D., Balas, A., König, P., Graff, G. R., & Madsen, R. W. (2003). Internet-enabled interactive multimedia asthma education program: A randomized trial. *Pediatrics, 111*, 503–510.

Kruse, W., & Weber, E. (1990). dynamics of drug regimen compliance – it's assessment by microprocessor-based monitoring. *European Journal of Clinical Pharmacology, 38*, 561–565.

Kuhn, T. S. (1970). *The structure of scientific revolutions* (2nd ed.). Chicago: The University of Chicago Press.

Kulik, J. A., & Carlino, P. (1987). The effect of verbal commitment and treatment choice on medication compliance in a pediatric setting. *Journal of Behavioral Medicine, 10*, 367–376.

Kumar, P. J., Walker-Smith, J., Milla, P., Harris, G., Colyer, J., & Halliday, R. (1988). The teenage coeliac: Follow up study of 102 patients. *Archives of Disease in Childhood, 63*, 916–920.

Kumar, V. S., Wentzell, K. J., Mikkelsen, T., Pentland, A., & Laffel, L. M. (2004). The DAILY (Daily Automated Intensive Log for Youth) trial: A wireless, portable system to improve adherence and glycemic control in youth with diabetes. *Diabetes Technology & Therapeutics, 6*, 445–453.

Kurtin, P. S., Landgraf, J. M., & Abetz, L. (1994). Patient-based health status measurements in pediatric dialysis: Expanding the assessment of outcome. *American Journal of Kidney Disease, 24*, 376–382.

Kvien, T. K., & Reimers, S. (1983). Drug handling and patient compliance in an outpatient paediatric trial. *Journal of Clinical & Hospital Pharmacy, 8*, 251–257.

Laffel, L. M. B., Vangsness, L., Connell, A., Goebel-Fabbri, A., Butler, D., & Anderson, B. J. (2003). Impact of ambulatory, family-focused teamwork intervention on glycemic control in youth with type 1 diabetes. *Journal of Pediatrics, 142*, 409–416.

La Greca, A. M. (1990). Issues in adherence with pediatric regimens. *Journal of Pediatric Psychology, 15*, 423–436.

La Greca, A. M., Auslander, W. F., Greca, P., Spetter, D., Fisher, E. B., & Santiago, J. V. (1995). I get by with a little help from my family and friends: Adolescents' support for diabetes care. *Journal of Pediatric Psychology, 20*, 449–476.

La Greca, A. M., Follansbee, D., & Skyler, J. S. (1990). Developmental and behavioral aspects of diabetes management in youngsters. *Children's Health Care, 19*, 132–139.

La Greca, A. M., Swales, T., Klemp, S., & Madigan, S. (1988). Self care behaviors among adolescents with diabetes. *Proceedings of the 9th annual sessions of the Society of Behavioral Medicine*, A42.

Lancaster, D., Lennard, L., & Lilleyman, J. S. (1997). Profile of non-compliance in lymphoblastic leukaemia. *Archives of Disease in Childhood, 76*, 365–366.

Landgraf, J. M., Abetz, L., & Ware, J. E. (1996). *The CHQ user's manual* (1st ed.). Boston: The Health Institute, New England Medical Center.

Lansky, S. B., Smith, S. D., Cairns, N. U., & Cairns, G. F. (1983). Psychological correlates of compliance. *The American Journal of Pediatric Hematology/Oncology, 5*, 87–92.

Lau, R. C. W., Matsui, D., Greenberg, M., & Koren, G. (1998). Electronic measurement of compliance with mercaptopurine in pediatric patients with acute lymphoblastic leukemia. *Medical and Pediatric Oncology, 30*, 85–90.

Lavigne, J. V., & Faier-Routman, J. (1992). Psychological adjustment to pediatric physical disorders: A meta-analytic review. *Journal of Pediatric Psychology, 17*, 133–157.

Lawson, M. L., Cohen, N., Richardson, C., & Orrbine, E. (2005). A randomized trial of regular standardized telephone contact by a diabetes nurse educator in adolescents with poor diabetes control. *Pediatric Diabetes, 6*, 32–40.

LeBaron, S., Zeltzer, L. K., Ratner, P., & Kniker, W. T. (1985). A controlled study of education for improving compliance with cromolyn sodium (intal®): The importance of physician-patient communication. *Annals of Allergy, 55*, 811–818.

Lee, W. C., Balu, S., Cobden, D., Joshi, A. V., & Pashos, C. L. (2006). Prevalence and economic consequences of medication adherence in diabetes: A systematic literature review. *Managed Care Interface, 19*, 31–41.

Lehane, E., & McCarthy, G. (2007). Intentional and unintentional medication non-adherence: A comprehensive framework for clinical research and practice? *International Journal of Nursing Studies, 44*, 1468–1477.

Lewandowski, A., & Drotar, D. (2007). The relationship between parent-reported social support and adherence to medical treatment in families of adolescents with type 1 diabetes. *Journal of Pediatric Psychology, 32*, 427–436.

Lewis, C. E., Rachelefsky, G., Lewis, M. A., de la Sota, A., & Kaplan, M. (1984). A randomized trial of A.C.T. (Asthma Care Training) for kids. *Pediatrics, 74*, 478–486.

Lipsey, M. W., & Wilson, D. B. (2001). *Practical meta-analysis*. Thousand Oaks, CA: Sage Publications.

Litt, I. F., & Cuskey, W. R. (1981). Compliance with salicylate therapy in adolescents with juvenile rheumatoid arthritis. *American Journal of Diseases of Children, 135*, 434–436.

Litt, I. F., Cuskey, W. R., & Rosenberg, A. (1982). Role of self-esteem and autonomy in determining medication compliance among adolescents with juvenile rheumatoid arthritis. *Pediatrics, 69*, 15–17.

Logan, D., Zelikovsky, N., Labay, L., & Spergel, J. (2003). The illness management survey: Identifying adolescents' perceptions of barriers to adherence. *Journal of Pediatric Psychology, 28*, 383–392.

Lorenz, R. A., Christensen, N. K., & Pichert, J. W. (1985). Diet-related knowledge, skill, and adherence among children with insulin-dependent diabetes mellitus. *Pediatrics, 75*, 872–876.

Lovell, D. J., Giannini, E. H., & Brewer, E. J. (1984). Time course of response to nonsteroidal antiinflammatory drugs in juvenile rheumatoid arthritis. *Arthritis and Rheumatism, 27*, 1433–1437.

Lowe, K., & Lutzker, J. R. (1979). Increasing compliance to a medical regimen with a juvenile diabetic. *Behavior Therapy, 10*, 57–64.

Lutfey, K. E., & Wishner, W. J. (1999). Beyond "compliance" is "adherence". *Diabetes Care, 22*, 635–639.

Mackner, L. M., & Crandall, W. V. (2005). Oral medication adherence in pediatric inflammatory bowel disease. *Inflammatory Bowel Diseases, 11*, 1006–1012.

Magee, J. C., Bucuvalas, J. C., Farmer, D. G., Harmon, W. E., Hulbert-Shearon, T. E., & Mendeloff, E. N. (2004). Pediatric transplantation. *American Journal of Transplantation, 4*(Suppl. 9), 54–71.

Magrab, P. R., & Papadopoulou, Z. L. (1977). The effect of a token economy on dietary compliance for children on hemodialysis. *Journal of Applied Behavior Analysis, 10*, 573–578.

Mahoney, M. J. (1974). *Cognition and behavior modification*. Cambridge, MA: Ballinger.

Maikranz, J. M., Steele, R. G., Dreyer, M. L., Stratman, A. C., & Bovaird, J. A. (2007). The relationship of hope and illness-related uncertainty to emotional adjustment and adherence among pediatric renal and liver transplant recipients. *Journal of Pediatric Psychology, 32*, 571–581.

Maiman, L. A., Becker, M. H., Liptak, G. S., Nazarian, L. F., & Rounds, K. A. (1988). Improving pediatricians' compliance-enhancing practices: A randomized trial. *American Journal of Diseases of Children, 142*, 773–779.

Marhefka, S. L., Tepper, V. J., Farley, J. J., Sleasman, J. W., & Mellins, C. A. (2006). Brief report: Assessing adherence to pediatric antiretroviral regimens using the 24-hour recall interview. *Journal of Pediatric Psychology, 31*, 989–994.

Mariani, P., Viti, M. G., Montouri, M., La Vecchia, A., Cipolletta, E., Calvani, L., et al. (1998). The gluten-free diet: A nutritional risk factor for adolescents with celiac disease? *Journal of Pediatric Gastroenterology and Nutrition, 27*, 519–523.

Marosi, A., & Stiesmeyer, J. (2001). Improving pediatric asthma patient outcomes by incorporation of effective interventions. *Journal of Asthma, 38*, 681–690.

Martin, S., Elliot-DeSorbo, D. K., Wolters, P. L., Toledo-Tamula, M. A., Roby, G., Zeichner, S., et al. (2007). Patient, caregiver and regimen characteristics associated with adherence to highly active antiretroviral therapy among HIV-infected children and adolescents. *Pediatric Infectious Disease Journal, 26*, 61–67.

Mash, E. J., & Terdal, L. G. (1988). Behavioral assessment of child and family disturbance. In E. J. Mash & L. G. Terdal (Eds.), *Behavioral assessment of childhood disorders* (2nd ed., pp. 3–65). New York: Guilford.

Matsui, D., Barron, A., & Rieder, M. J. (1996). Assessment of the palatability of antistaphylococcal antibiotics in pediatric volunteers. *The Annals of Pharmacotherapy, 30*, 586–588.

Matsui, D., Hermann, C., Braudo, M., Ito, S., Olivieri, N., & Koren, G. (1992). Clinical use of the medication event monitoring system: A new window into pediatric compliance. *Clinical Pharmacology and Therapeutics, 52*, 102–103.

Matsuyama, J. R., Mason, B. J., & Jue, S. G. (1993). Pharmacists' interventions using an electronic medication-event monitoring device's adherence data versus pill counts. *The Annals of Pharmacotherapy, 27*, 851–855.

Mattar, M. F., Marklein, J., & Yaffe, S. J. (1975). Pharmaceutic factors affecting pediatric compliance. *Pediatrics, 55,* 101–108.

McCaul, K. D., Glasgow, R. E., & Schafer, L. C. (1987). Diabetes regimen behaviors: Predicting adherence. *Medical Care, 25,* 868–881.

McCormick, M. C., Stemmler, M. M., & Athreya, B. H. (1986). The impact of childhood rheumatic diseases on the family. *Arthritis & Rheumatism, 29,* 872–879.

McGrath, P. A. (1990). *Pain in children: Nature, assessment and treatment.* New York: Guilford.

McLinn, S. E., McCarty, J. M., Perrotta, R., Pichichero, M. E., & Reindenberg, B. E. (1995). Multicenter controlled trial comparing ceftibuten with amoxicillin/clavulantae in the empiric treatment of acute otitis media. *Pediatric Infectious Disease Journal, 14,* 5108–5114.

McPherson, A. C., Glazebrook, C., Forster, D., James, C., & Smyth, A. (2006). A randomized, controlled trial of an interactive educational computer package for children with asthma. *Pediatrics, 117,* 1046–1054.

McQuaid, E. L., Kopel, S. J., Klein, R. B., & Fritz, G. K. (2003). Medication adherence in pediatric asthma: Reasoning, responsibility, and behavior. *Journal of Pediatric Psychology, 28,* 323–333.

McQuaid, E. L., Walders, N., Kopel, S. J., Fritz, G. K., & Klinnert, M. D. (2005). Pediatric asthma management in the family context: The family asthma management system scale. *Journal of Pediatric Psychology, 30,* 492–502.

Meade, C. D., & Smith, C. F. (1991). Readability formulas: Cautions and criteria. *Patient Education and Counseling, 17,* 153–158.

Meichenbaum, D., & Turk, D. C. (1987). *Facilitating treatment adherence: A practitioner's guidebook.* New York: Plenum.

Mellins, C. A., Brackis-Cott, E., Dolezal, C., & Abrams, E. J. (2004). The role of psychosocial and family factors in adherence to antiretroviral treatment in human immunodeficiency virus-infected children. *Pediatric Infectious Disease Journal, 23,* 1035–1041.

Méndez, F. J., & Beléndez, M. (1997). Effects of a behavioral intervention on treatment adherence and stress management in adolescents with IDDM. *Diabetes Care, 20,* 1370–1375.

Milgrom, H., Bender, B., Ackerson, L., Bowry, P., Smith, B., & Rand, C. (1996). Noncompliance and treatment failure in children with asthma. *Journal of Allergy & Clinical Immunology, 98,* 1051–1057.

Miller, K. A. (1982). Theophylline compliance in adolescent patients with chronic asthma. *Journal of Adolescent Health Care, 3,* 177–179.

Miller, V. A., & Drotar, D. (2003). Discrepancies between mother and adolescent perceptions of diabetes-related decision-making autonomy and their relationship to diabetes-related conflict and adherence to treatment. *Journal of Pediatric Psychology, 28,* 265–274.

Miller, V. A., & Drotar, D. (2007). Decision-making competence and adherence to treatment in adolescents with diabetes. *Journal of Pediatric Psychology, 32,* 178–188.

Millstein, S. G., Petersen, A. C., & Nightingale, E. O. (1993). *Promoting the health of adolescents: New directions for the twenty-first century.* New York: Oxford University Press.

Mitchell, W. G., Scheier, L. M., & Baker, S. A. (2000). Adherence to treatment in children with epilepsy: Who follows "doctor's orders"? *Epilepsia, 41,* 1616–1625.

Modi, A. C., Crosby, L. E., Guilfoyle, S. M., Lemanek, K. L., Witherspoon, D., & Mitchell, M. J. (2009). Barriers to treatment adherence for pediatric patients with sickle cell disease and their families. *Children's Health Care, 38,* 107–122.

Modi, A. C., Lim, C. S., Yu, N., Geller, D., Wagner, M. H., & Quittner, A. L. (2006). A multi-method assessment of treatment adherence for children with cystic fibrosis. *Journal of Cystic Fibrosis, 5,* 177–185.

Modi, A. C., Morita, D. A., & Glauser, T. A. (2008). One-month adherence in children with new-onset epilepsy: White-coat compliance does not occur. *Pediatrics, 121,* e1–e6.

Modi, A. C., & Quittner, A. L. (2006a). Barriers to treatment adherence for children with cystic fibrosis and asthma: What gets in the way? *Journal of Pediatric Psychology, 31,* 846–858.

Modi, A. C., & Quittner, A. L. (2006b). Utilizing computerized phone diary procedures to assess health behaviors in family and social contexts. *Children's Health Care, 35,* 29–45.

Montaño, D. E., Kasprzyk, K. D., & Taplin, S. H. (1997). The theory of reasoned action and the theory of planned behavior. In K. Glanz, F. Lewis, & B. K. Rimer (Eds.), *Health behavior and health education: Theory, research, and practice* (2nd ed., pp. 85–112). San Francisco: Jossey-Bass.

Mora, S., Barera, G., Beccio, S., Menni, L., Proverbio, M. C., Bianchi, C., et al. (2001). A prospective, longitudinal study of the long-term effect of treatment on bone density in children with celiac disease. *The Journal of Pediatrics, 139*, 516–521.

Morse, E. V., Simon, P. M., & Balson, P. M. (1993). Using experimental training to enhance health professionals' awareness of patient compliance issues. *Academic Medicine, 68*, 693–697.

Murphy, M. S., Sood, M., & Johnson, T. (2002). Use of the lactose H_2 breath test to monitor mucosal healing in coeliac disease. *Acta Paediatrica, 91*, 141–144.

Myers, R. S., & Roth, D. L. (1997). Perceived benefits of and barriers to exercise and stage of exercise adoption in young adults. *Health Psychology, 16*, 277–283.

Naar-King, S., Frey, M., Harris, M., & Arfken, C. (2005). Measuring adherence to treatment of paediatric HIV/AIDS. *AIDS Care, 17*, 345–349.

Naar-King, S., Idalski, A., Ellis, D., Frey, M., Templin, T., Cunningham, P. B., et al. (2006). Gender differences in adherence and metabolic control in urban youth with poorly controlled type 1 diabetes: The mediating role of mental health symptoms. *Journal of Pediatric Psychology, 31*, 793–802.

National Asthma Education and Prevention Program. (1997). *Expert panel report 2: Guidelines for the diagnosis and management of asthma.* Bethesda, MD: National Institutes of Health (Publication No. 97–4051).

O'Donohue, W., & Krasner, L. (1995). Theories in behavior therapy: Philosophical and historical contexts. In W. O'Donohue & L. Krasner (Eds.), *Theories of behavior therapy: Exploring behavior change* (pp. 1–22). Washington DC: American Psychological Association.

Oermann, M. H., Gerich, J., Ostosh, L., & Zaleski, S. (2003). Evaluation of asthma websites for patient and parent education. *Journal of Pediatric Nursing, 18*, 389–396.

O'Leary, A. (1985). Self-efficacy and health. *Behavior Research and Therapy, 23*, 437–451.

O'Leary, A. (1992). Self-efficacy and health: Behavioral and stress-physiological mediation. *Cognitive Therapy and Research, 16*, 229–245.

Oliva-Hemker, M. M., Abadom, V., Cuffari, C., & Thompson, R. E. (2007). Nonadherence with thiopurine immunomodulator and mesalamine medications in children with Crohn disease. *Journal of Pediatric Gastroenterology and Nutrition, 44*, 180–184.

Olivieri, N. F., Matsui, D., Hermann, C., & Koren, G. (1991). Compliance assessed by the medication event monitoring systems. *Archives of Disease in Childhood, 66*, 1399–1402.

Olivieri, N. F., & Vichinsky, E. P. (1998). Hydroxyurea in children with sickle cell disease: Impact on splenic function and compliance with therapy. *Journal of Pediatric Hematology/Oncology, 20*, 26–31.

O'Neill, R. E., Horner, R. H., Albin, R. W., Storey, K., & Sprague, J. R. (1990). *Functional analysis of problem behavior: A practical assessment guide.* Sycamore, IL: Sycamore Publishing.

Ooi, C. Y., Bohane, T. D., Lee, D., Naidoo, D., & Day, A. S. (2007). Thiopurine metabolite monitoring in paediatric inflammatory bowel disease. *Alimentary Pharmacology and Therapeutics, 25*, 941–947.

Osterberg, L., & Blaschke, T. (2005). Drug therapy: Adherence to medication. *The New England Journal of Medicine, 353*, 487–498.

Pai, A. L. H., Drotar, D., & Kodish, E. (2008). Correspondence between objective and subjective reports of adherence among adolescents with acute lymphoblastic leukemia. *Children's Health Care.*

Palermo, T. M., Long, A. C., Lewandowski, A. S., Drotar, D., Quittner, A. L., & Walker, L. S. (2008). Evidence-based assessment of health-related quality of life and functional impairment in pediatric psychology. *Journal of Pediatric Psychology, 33*, 983–996.

Palermo, T. M., Valenzuela, D., & Stork, P. P. (2004). A randomized trial of electronic versus paper pain diaries in children: Impact on compliance, accuracy, and acceptability. *Pain, 107*, 213–219.

Parcel, G. S., Swank, P. R., Mariotto, M. J., Bartholomew, L. K., Czyzewski, D. I., Sockrider, M. M., et al. (1994). Self-management of cystic fibrosis: A structural model for educational and behavioral variables. *Social Science & Medicine, 38*, 1307–1315.

Park, D. C., & Kidder, D. P. (1996). Prospective memory and medication adherence. In M. Brandimonte, G. O. Einstein, & M. A. McDaniel (Eds.), *Prospective memory: Theory and applications* (pp. 369–390). Mahwah, NJ: Lawrence Erlbaum Associates.

Passero, M. A., Remor, B., & Salomon, J. (1981). Patient-reported compliance with cystic fibrosis therapy. *Clinical Pediatrics, 20*, 264–268.

Patino, A. M., Sanchez, J., Eidson, M., & Delamater, A. M. (2005). Health beliefs and regimen adherence in minority adolescents with type 1 diabetes. *Journal of Pediatric Psychology, 30*, 503–512.

Patrick, D. L., Edwards, T. C., & Topolski, T. D. (2002). Adolescent quality of life, Part II: Initial validation of a new instrument. *Journal of Adolescence, 25*, 287–300.

Patterson, J. M. (1985). Critical factors affecting family compliance with home treatment for children with cystic fibrosis. *Family Relations, 34*, 79–89.

Patwari, A. K., Anand, V. K., Kapur, G., & Narayan, S. (2003). Clinical and nutritional profile of children with celiac disease. *Indian Pediatrics, 40*, 337–342.

Penkower, L., Dew, M. A., Ellis, D., Sereika, S. M., Kitutu, J. M. M., & Shapiro, R. (2003). Psychological distress and adherence to the medical regimen among adolescent renal transplant recipients. *American Journal of Transplantation, 3*, 1418–1425.

Perrin, E. C., Stein, R. E. K., & Drotar, D. (1991). Cautions in using the child behavior checklist: Observations based on research about children with a chronic illness. *Journal of Pediatric Psychology, 16*, 411–421.

Peterson, A. M., Takiya, L., & Finley, R. (2003). Meta-analysis of trials of interventions to improve medication adherence. *American Journal of Health-Systems Pharmacy, 60*, 657–665.

Pew Internet & American Life Project (2006). *Online health search 2006.* Washington, DC: Pew Foundation.

Phipps, S., & DeCuir-Whalley, S. (1990). Adherence issues in pediatric bone marrow transplantation. *Journal of Pediatric Psychology, 15*, 459–475.

Phipps, S., Hinds, P. S., Channell, S., & Bell, G. L. (1994). Measurement of behavioral, affective, and somatic responses to pediatric bone marrow transplantation: Development of the BASES scale. *Journal of Pediatric Oncology Nursing, 11*, 109–117.

Pichichero, M. E., Disney, F. A., Aronovitz, G. H., Talpey, W. B., Green, J. L., & Francis, A. B. (1987). Randomized, single-blind evaluation of cefadroxil and phenoxy-methylpenicillin in the treatment of streptococcal pharyngitis. *Antimicrobial Agents & Chemotherapy, 31*, 903–906.

Pieper, K. B., Rapoff, M. A., Purviance, M. R., & Lindsley, C. B. (1989). Improving compliance with prednisone therapy in pediatric patients with rheumatic disease. *Arthritis Care & Research, 2*, 132–135.

Poppen, R. L. (1989). Some clinical implications of rule-governed behavior. In S. C. Hayes (Ed.), *Rule-governed behavior: Cognition, contingencies, and instructional control* (pp. 325–357). New York: Plenum.

Popper, K. R. (1963). *Conjectures and refutations.* New York: Harper & Row.

Powers, S. W., Jones, J. S., Perguson, K. S., Piazza-Waggoner, C., Daines, C., & Acton, J. D. (2005). Randomized clinical trial of behavioral and nutrition treatment to improve energy intake and growth in toddlers and preschoolers with cystic fibrosis. *Pediatrics, 116*, 1442–1450.

Prochaska, J. O. (1979). *Systems of psychotherapy: A transtheoretical analysis.* Homewood, IL: Dorsey.

Prochaska, J. O., & DiClemente, C. C. (1983). Stages and processes of self-change of smoking: Toward an integrative model of change. *Journal of Consulting and Clinical Psychology, 51*, 390–395.

Prochaska, J. O., DiClemente, C. C., & Norcross, J. C. (1992). In search of how people change: Applications to addictive behaviors. *American Psychologist, 47*, 1102–1114.

Prochaska, J. O., Johnson, S., & Lee, P. (2009). The transtheoretical model of behavior change. In S. A. Shumaker, J. K. Ockene, & K. A. Riekert (Eds.), *The handbook of health behavior change* (3rd ed., pp. 59–83). New York: Springer.

Prochaska, J. O., Redding, C. A., & Evers, K. E. (1997). The transtheoretical model and stages of change. In K. Glanz, F. M. Lewis, & B. K. Rimer (Eds.), *Health behavior and health education: Theory, research, and practice* (2nd ed., pp. 60–84). San Francisco: Jossey-Bass.

Prochaska, J. O., Velicer, W. F., Rossi, J. S., Goldstein, M. G., Marcus, B. H., Rakowski, W. et al., (1994). Stages of change and decisional balance for 12 problem behaviors. *Health Psychology, 13*, 39–46.

Quittner, A. L., Buu, A., Messer, M. A., Modi, A. C., & Watrous, M. (2005). Development and validation of the cystic fibrosis questionnaire in the United States: A health-related quality-of-life measure for cystic fibrosis. *Chest, 128*, 2347–2354.

Quittner, A. L., Espelage, D. L., Ievers-Landis, C., & Drotar, D. (2000). Measuring adherence to medical treatments in childhood chronic illness: Considering multiple methods and sources of information. *Journal of Clinical Psychology in Medical Settings, 7*, 41–54.

Quittner, A. L., Modi, A. C., Lemanek, K. L., Ievers-Landis, C. E., & Rapoff, M. A. (2008). Evidence-based assessment of adherence to medical treatments in pediatric psychology. *Journal of Pediatric Psychology, 33*, 916–936.

Quittner, A. L., & Opipari, L. C. (1994). Differential treatment of siblings: Interview and diary analyses comparing two family contexts. *Child Development, 65*, 800–814.

Rabinovich, M., MacKenzie, R., Brazeau, M., & Marks, M. I. (1973). Treatment of streptococcal pharyngitis. I. Clinical evaluation. *Canadian Medical Association Journal, 108*, 1271–1274.

Radius, S. M., Marshall, H. B., Rosenstock, I. M., Drachman, R. H., Schuberth, K. C., & Teets, K. C. (1978). Factors influencing mothers' compliance with a medication regimen for asthmatic children. *Journal of Asthma Research, 15*, 133–149.

Rand, C. S. (2000). "I took the medicine like you told me, doctor": Self-report of adherence with medical regimens. In A. A. Stone, J. S. Turkkan, C. A. Bachrach, J. B. Jobe, H. S. Kurtzman, & V. S. Cain (Eds.), *The science of self-report: Implications for research and practice* (pp. 257–276). Mahwah, NJ: Lawrence Erlbaum Associates.

Rand, C. S., & Wise, R. A. (1994). Measuring adherence to asthma medication regimens. *American Journal of Critical Care Medicine, 149*, 569–576.

Rapoff, M. A. (1989). Compliance with treatment regimens for pediatric rheumatic diseases. *Arthritis Care & Research, 2*(Suppl.), 40–47.

Rapoff, M. A. (1996, Summer). Why comply? Theories in pediatric medical adherence research. *Progress Notes: Newsletter of the Society of Pediatric Psychology, 20*(6), 3–4.

Rapoff, M. A. (1997). *Helping children follow their medical treatment program: Guidelines for parents of children with rheumatic diseases.* Available from the author, University of Kansas Medical Center, Department of Pediatrics, 3901 Rainbow Blvd., Kansas City, KS 66160–7330.

Rapoff, M. A. (1999). *Adherence to pediatric medical regimens.* New York: Kluwer/Plenum.

Rapoff, M. A. (2000). Facilitating adherence to medical regimens for pediatric rheumatic diseases: Primary, secondary, and tertiary prevention. In D. Drotar (Ed.), *Promoting adherence to medical treatment in chronic childhood illness: Concepts, methods, and interventions* (pp. 329–345). Mahwah, NJ: Lawrence Erlbaum Associates.

Rapoff, M. A., & Barnard, M. U. (1991). Compliance with pediatric medical regimens. In J. A. Cramer & B. Spilker (Eds.), *Patient compliance in medical practice and clinical trials* (pp. 73–98). New York: Raven Press.

Rapoff, M. A., Belmont, J., Lindsley, C., Olson, N., Morris, J., & Padur, J. (2002). Prevention of nonadherence to nonsteroidal anti-inflammatory medications for newly diagnosed patients with juvenile rheumatoid arthritis. *Health Psychology, 21*, 620–623.

Rapoff, M. A., Belmont, J. M., Lindsley, C. B., & Olson, N. Y. (2005). Electronically monitored adherence to medications by newly diagnosed patients with juvenile rheumatoid arthritis.
Arthritis Care & Research, 53, 905–910.

Rapoff, M. A., & Christophersen, E. R. (1982). Compliance of pediatric patients with
medical regimens: A review and evaluation. In R. B. Stuart (Ed.), *Adherence, compliance, and generalization in behavioral medicine* (pp. 79–124). New York: Brunner/
Mazel.

Rapoff, M. A., Lindsley, C. B., & Christophersen, E. R. (1984). Improving compliance with medical regimens: Case study with juvenile rheumatoid arthritis. *Archives of Physical Medicine &
Rehabilitation, 65*, 267–269.

Rapoff, M. A., Lindsley, C. B., & Christophersen, E. R. (1985). Parent perceptions of problems
experienced by their children in complying with treatments for juvenile rheumatoid arthritis.
Archives of Physical Medicine & Rehabilitation, 66, 427–430.

Rapoff, M. A., Purviance, M. R., & Lindsley, C. B. (1988a). Educational and behavioral strategies
for improving medication compliance in juvenile rheumatoid arthritis. *Archives of Physical
Medicine and Rehabilitation. 69*, 439–441.

Rapoff, M. A., Purviance, M. R., & Lindsley, C. B. (1988b). Improving medication compliance
for juvenile rheumatoid arthritis and its effect on clinical outcome: A single-subject analysis.
Arthritis Care & Research, 1, 12–16.

Rapoff, M. A., & Stark, L. (2008). *Journal of Pediatric Psychology* Statement of Purpose: Section
on single-subject studies. *Journal of Pediatric Psychology, 33*, 16–21.

Rashid, M., Cranney, A., Zarkadas, M., Graham, I. D., Switzer, C., Case, S., et al., (2005). Celiac
disease: Evaluation of the diagnosis and dietary compliance in Canadian children. *Pediatrics,
116*, 754–759.

Reddington, C. Cohen, J., Baldillo, A., Toye, M., Smith, D., Kneut, C., et al., (2000). Adherence to
medication regimens among children with human immunodeficiency virus infection. *Pediatric
Infectious Disease Journal, 19*, 1148–1153.

Reynolds, L. A., Johnson, S. B., & Silverstein, J. (1990). Assessing daily diabetes management by
24-hour recall interview: The validity of children's reports. *Journal of Pediatric Psychology,
15*, 493–509.

Riegler, H. C., & Baer, D. M. (1989). A developmental analysis of rule-following. *Advances in
Child Development and Behavior, 21*, 191–219.

Riekert, K. A., & Rand, C. S. (2002). Electronic monitoring of medication adherence: When is
high-tech best? *Journal of Clinical Psychology in Medical Settings, 9*, 25–34.

Ritterband, L. M., Gonder-Frederick, L. A., Cox, D. J., Clifton, A. D., West, R. W., & Borowitz,
S. M. (2003). Internet interventions: In review, in use, and into the future. *Professional
Psychology: Research and Practice, 34*, 527–534.

Roberts, G. M., Wheeler, G., Tucker, N. C., Hackler, C., Young, K., Maples, H. D, et al., (2004).
Nonadherence with pediatric human immunodeficiency virus therapy as medical neglect.
Pediatrics, 114, e346–e353.

Roberts, M. C., & Wallander, J. L. (1992). Family issues in pediatric psychology: An overview.
In M. C. Roberts & J. L. Wallander (Eds.), *Family issues in pediatric psychology* (pp. 1–24).
Mahwah, NJ: Erlbaum.

Rock, D. L., Bransford, J. D., Maisto, S. A., & Morey, L. (1987). The study of clinical judgement:
An ecological approach. *Clinical Psychology Review, 7*, 645–661.

Rodewald, L. E., Maiman, L. A., Foye, H. R., Borch, R. F., & Forbes, G. B. (1989). Deuterium
oxide as a tracer for measurement of compliance in pediatric clinical drug trials. *Journal of
Pediatrics, 114*, 885–891.

Rodrigues, A. F., Johnson, T., Davies, P., & Murphy, M. S. (2007). Does polymeric formula
improve adherence to liquid diet therapy in children with active Crohn's disease? *Archives
of Disease in Childhood, 92*, 767–770.

Rosen, C. S. (2000). Is the sequencing of change processes by stage consistent across health
problems? A meta-analysis. *Health Psychology, 19*, 593–604.

Rosenbaum, P., Cadman, D., & Kirpalani, H. (1990). Pediatrics: Assessing quality of life. In B. Spilker (Ed.), *Qualify of life assessments in clinical trials* (pp. 205–215). New York: Raven.

Rosenstock, I. M. (1974). Historical origins of the health belief model. *Health Education Monographs, 2*, 328–335.

Rosenthal, R. (1991). *Meta-analytic procedures for social research*. Thousand Oaks, CA: Sage Publications.

Roter, D. L., Hall, J. A., Merisca, R., Nordstrom, B., Cretin, D., & Svarstad, B. (1998). Effectiveness of interventions to improve compliance: A meta-analysis. *Medical Care, 36*, 1138–1161.

Roth, H. P. (1987). Current perspectives: Ten year update on patient compliance research. *Patient Education and Counseling, 10*, 107–116.

Rowbothan, M. C. (2001). What is a 'clinically meaningful' reduction in pain? *Pain, 94*, 131–132.

Rubio, A., Cox, C., & Weintraub, M. (1992). Prediction of diltiazem plasma concentration curves from limited measurements using compliance data. *Clinical Pharmacokinetics, 22*, 238–246.

Rubin, D. H., Leventhal, J. M., Sadock, R. T., Letovsky, E., Schottland, P., Clemente, et al., (1986). Educational intervention by computer in childhood asthma: A randomized clinical trial testing the use of a new teaching intervention in childhood asthma. *Pediatrics, 77*, 1–10.

Rudd, P. (1993). The measurement of compliance: Medication taking. In M. A. Krasnegor, L. Epstein, S. B. Johnson, & S. J. Yaffe (Eds.), *Developmental aspects of health compliance behavior* (pp. 185–213). Hillsdale, NJ: Lawrence Erlbaum.

Ruggiero, L. (2000). Helping people with diabetes change behavior: From theory to practice. *Diabetes Spectrum, 13*, 125–132.

Ruggiero, L., & Prochaska, J. O. (1993). Readiness for change: Application of the transtheoretical model to diabetes. *Diabetes Spectrum, 6*, 21–60.

Ryle, G. (1949). *The concept of mind*. Chicago: The University of Chicago Press.

Saadah, O. I., Zacharin, M., O'Callaghan, A., Oliver, M. R., & Catto-Smith, A. G. (2004). Effect of gluten-free diet and adherence on growth and diabetic control in diabetics with coeliac disease. *Archives of Disease in Childhood, 89*, 871–876.

Sanz, E. J. (2003). Concordance and children's use of medicines. *British Medical Journal, 327*, 858–860.

Satin, W., La Greca, A. M., Zigo, M. A., & Skyler, J. S. (1989). Diabetes in adolescence: Effects of multifamily group intervention and parent simulation of diabetes. *Journal of Pediatric Psychology, 14*, 259–275.

Schafer, L. C., Glasgow, R. E., & McCaul, K. D. (1982). Increasing the adherence of diabetic adolescents. *Journal of Behavioral Medicine, 5*, 353–362.

Schlösser, M., & Havermans, G. (1992). A self-efficacy scale for children and adolescents with asthma: Construction and validation. *Journal of Asthma, 29*, 99–108.

Schmidt, L. E., Klover, R. V., Arfken, C. L., Delamater, A. M., & Hobson, D. (1992). Compliance with dietary prescriptions in children and adolescents with insulin-dependent diabetes mellitus. *Journal of the American Dietetic Association, 92*, 567–570.

Schwartz, R. H., Rodriques, W. J., & Grundfast, K. M. (1981). Pharmacologic compliance with antibiotic therapy for acute otitis media: Influence on subsequent middle ear effusion. *Pediatrics, 68*, 619–622.

Schwartz-Lookinland, S., McKeever, L. C., & Saputo, M. (1989). Compliance with antibiotic regimens in Hispanic mothers. *Patient Education & Counseling, 13*, 171–182.

Schwarzer, R., & Fuchs, R. (1995). Changing risk behaviors and adopting health behaviors: The role of self-efficacy beliefs. In A. Bandura (Ed.), *Self-efficacy in changing societies* (pp. 259–288). New York: Cambridge University Press.

Selimoglu, M. A., Altinkaynak, S., Ertekin, V., & Akcay, F. (2006). Serum ghrelin levels in children with celiac disease. *Journal of Clinical Gastroenterology, 40*, 191–194.

Sergis-Davenport, E., & Varni, J. W. (1983). Behavioral assessment and management of adherence to factor replacement therapy in hemophilia. *Journal of Pediatric Psychology, 8*, 367–377.

Serrano-Ikkos, E., Lask, B., Whitehead, B., & Eisler, I. (1998). Incomplete adherence after pediatric heart and heart-lung transplantation. *Journal of Heart & Lung Transplantation, 17*, 1177–1183.

Shellmer, D. A., & Zelikovsky, N. (2007). The challenges of using medication event monitoring technology with pediatric transplant patients. *Pediatric Transplantation, 11*, 422–428

Shemesh, E., Lurie, S., Stuber, M. L., Emre, S., Patel, Y., Vohra, P, et al., (2000). A pilot study of posttraumatic stress and nonadherence in pediatric liver transplant recipients. *Pediatrics, 105*, e29.

Shemesh, E., Shneider, B. L., Savitzky, J. K., Arnott, L., Gondolesi, G. E., Krieger, N. R., et al., (2004). Medication adherence in pediatric and adolescent liver transplant recipients. *Pediatrics, 113*, 825–832.

Shingadia, D., Viani, R. M., Yogev, R., Binns, H., Danker, W. M., Spector, S. A., et al., (2000). Gastrostomy tube insertion for improvement of adherence to highly active antiretroviral therapy in pediatric patients with human immunodeficiency virus. *Pediatrics, 105*, e80.

Silverman, A. H., Hains, A. A., Davies, W. H., & Parton, E. (2003). A cognitive behavioral adherence intervention for adolescents with type 1 diabetes. *Journal of Clinical Psychology in Medical Settings, 10*, 119–127.

Simons, L. E., & Blount, R. L. (2007). Identifying barriers to medication adherence in adolescent transplant recipients. *Journal of Pediatric Psychology, 32*, 831–844.

Simmons, F .E. R., Gerstner, T. V., & Cheang, M. S. (1997). Tolerance to bronchoprotective effect of salmeterol in adolescents with exercise-induced asthma using concurrent inhaled glucocorticoid treatment. *Pediatrics, 99*, 655–659.

Singh, G., Athreya, B. H., Fries, J. F., & Goldsmith, D. P. (1994). Measurement of health status in children with juvenile rheumatoid arthritis. *Arthritis & Rheumatism, 37*, 1761–1769.

Singh, J. (1995). The readability of educational materials written for parents of children with attention-deficit hyperactivity disorder. *Journal of Child & Family Studies, 4*, 207–218.

Skinner, B. F. (1974). *About behaviorism.* New York: Knopf.

Slack, M. K., & Brooks, A. J. (1995). Medication management issues for adolescents with asthma. *American Journal of Health-System Pharmacy, 52*, 1417–1421.

Sly, R. M. (1988). Mortality from asthma in children, 1979–1984. *Annals of Allergy, 60*, 433–443.

Smith, M. (1985). The cost of noncompliance and the capacity of improved compliance to reduce health care expenditures. *Improving medication compliance: Proceedings of a symposium .* Washington, DC: The National Pharmaceutical Council.

Smith, N. A., Seale, J. P., Ley, P., Mellis, C. M., & Shaw, J. (1994). Better medication compliance is associated with improved control of childhood asthma. *Monaldi Archive of Chest Disease, 49*, 470–474.

Smith, N. A., Seale, J. P., Ley, P., Shaw, J., & Braes, P. U. (1986). Effects of intervention on medication compliance in children with asthma. *The Medical Journal of Australia, 144*, 119–122.

Smith, S. D., Rosen, D., Trueworthy, R. C., & Lowman, J. T. (1979). A reliable method for evaluating drug compliance in children with cancer. *Cancer, 43*, 169–173.

Smyth, A. R., & Judd, B. A. (1993). Compliance with antibiotic prophylaxis in urinary tract infection. *Archives of Diseases of Children, 38*, 235–236.

Snodgrass, S. R., Vedanarayanan, V. V., Parker, C. C., & Parks, B. R. (2001). Pediatric patients with undetectable anticonvulsant blood levels: Comparison with compliant patients. *Journal of Child Neurology, 16*, 164–168.

Snyder, J. (1987). Behavioral analysis and treatment of poor diabetic self-care and antisocial behavior: A single-subject experimental study. *Behavior Therapy, 18*, 251–263.

Socolar, R., Amaya-Jackson, L., Eron, L. D., Howard, B., Landsverk, J., & Evans, J. (1997). Research on discipline: The state of the art, deficits, and implications. *Archives of Pediatric & Adolescent Medicine, 151*, 758–760.

Sokol, M. C., McGuigan, K. A., Verbrugge, R. R., & Epstein, R. S. (2005). Impact of medication adherence on hospitalization risk and healthcare cost. *Medical Care, 43*, 521–530.

Spieth, L. E., & Harris, C. V. (1996). Assessment of health-related quality of life in children and adolescents: An integrative review. *Journal of Pediatric Psychology, 21*, 175–193.

Starr, M., Sawyer, S. M., Carlin, J. B., Powell, C. V. E., Newman, R. G., & Johnson, P. D. R. (1999). A novel approach to monitoring adherence to preventive therapy for tuberculosis in adolescence. *Journal of Paediatric Child Health, 35*, 350–354.

Starfield, B., Riley, A. W., & Green, B. F. (1999). *Manual for the child health and illness profile: Adolescent edition (CHIP-AE)*. Baltimore: The Johns Hopkins University.

Stark, L. J., Hommell, K. A., Mackner, L., Janicke, D. M., Davis, A. M., Pfefferkorn, M. et al., (2005a). Randomized trial comparing two methods of increasing dietary calcium intake in children with inflammatory bowel disease. *Journal of Pediatric Gastroenterology and Nutrition, 40*, 501–507.

Stark, L. J., Janicke, D. M., McGrath, A. M., Mackner, L. M., Hommel, K. A., & Lovell, D. (2005b). Prevention of osteoporosis: A randomized clinical trial to increase calcium intake in children with juvenile rheumatoid arthritis. *Journal of Pediatric Psychology, 30*, 377–386.

Stark, L. J., Mackner, L. M., Kessler, J. H., Opipari, L. C., & Quittner, A. L. (2002). Preliminary findings for calcium intake in children with cystic fibrosis following behavioral intervention for caloric intake. *Children's Health Care, 31*, 107–118.

Stark, L. J., Miller, S. T., Plienes, A. J., & Drabman, R. S.(1987). Behavioral contracting to increase chest physiotherapy: A study of a young cystic fibrosis patient. *Behavior Modification, 11*, 75–86.

Stark, L. J., Opipari, L. C., Spieth, L. E., Jelalian, E., Quittner, A. L., Higgins, L., et al., (2003). Contribution of behavior therapy to dietary treatment in cystic fibrosis: A randomized controlled study with 2-year follow-up. *Behavior Therapy, 34*, 237–258.

Stewart, S. M., Lee, P. W. H., Waller, D., Hughes, C. W., Low, L. C. K., Kennard, et al., (2003). A follow-up study of adherence and glycemic control among Hong Kong youths with diabetes. *Journal of Pediatric Psychology, 28*, 67–79.

Stinson, J. N., Kavanagh, T., Yamada, J., Gill, N., & Stevens, B. (2006). Systematic review of the psychometric properties, interpretability and feasibility of self-report pain intensity measures for use in clinical trials in children and adolescents. *Pain, 125*, 143–157.

Strecher, V. J., DeVellis, B. M., Becker, M. H., & Rosenstock, I. M. (1986). The role of self-efficacy in achieving health behavior change. *Health Education Quarterly, 13*, 73–91.

Strecher, V. J., & Rosenstock, I. M. (1997). The health belief model. In K. Glanz, F. M. Lewis, & B. K. Rimer (Eds.), *Health behavior and health education: Theory, research, and practice* (2nd ed., pp. 41–59). San Francisco: Jossey-Bass.

Stroebe, W., & Stroebe, M. S. (1995). *Social psychology and health*. Pacific Grove, CA: Brooks/Cole.

Stuber, M. (1993). Psychiatric aspects of organ transplantation in children and adolescents. *Organ Transplantation in Children and Adolescents, 34*, 379–387.

Sturmey, P. (1996). *Functional analysis in clinical psychology*. New York: Wiley, John & Sons.

Sublett, J. L., Pollard, S. J., Kadlec, G. J., & Karibo, J. M. (1979). Non-compliance in asthmatic children: A study of theophylline levels in a pediatric emergency room population. *Annals of Allergy, 43*, 95–97.

Tamaroff, M. H., Festa, R. S., Adesman, A. R., & Walco, G. A. (1992). Therapeutic adherence to oral medication regimens by adolescents with cancer. II. Clinical and psychological correlates. *Journal of Pediatrics, 120*, 812–817.

Taylor, W. R., & Newacheck, P. W. (1992). Impact of childhood asthma on health. *Pediatrics, 90*, 657–662.

Tebbi, C. K., Cumings, K. M., Kevon, M. A., Smith, L., Richards, M., & Mallon, J. (1986). Compliance of pediatric and adolescent cancer patients. *Cancer, 58*, 1179–1184.

Tebbi, C. K., Richards, M. E., Cummings, K. M., Zevon, M. A., & Mallon, J. C. (1988). The role of parent-adolescent concordance in compliance with cancer chemotherapy. *Adolescence, 28*, 599–611.

The Task Force for Compliance (1994). *Noncompliance with medications: An economic tragedy with important implications for health care reform.* Baltimore: National Pharmaceutical Council.

Thomas, A. M., Peterson, L., & Goldstein, D. (1997). Problem solving and diabetes regimen adherence by children and adolescents with IDDM in social pressure situations: A reflection of normal development. *Journal of Pediatric Psychology, 22*, 541–561.

Tinkelman, D. G., Vanderpool, G. E., Carroll, M. S., Page, E. G., & Spangler, D. L. (1980). Compliance differences following administration of theophylline at six-and twelve-hour intervals. *Annals of Allergy, 44*, 283–286.

Todd, J. T., & Morris, E. K. (1992). Case histories in the great power of steady misrepresentation. *American Psychologist, 47*, 1441–1453.

Tommasini, A., Not, T., Kiren, V., Baldas, V. Santon, D., Trevisiol, C., et al., (2004). Mass screening for coeliac disease using antihuman transglutaminase antibody assay. *Archives of Disease in Childhood, 89*, 512–515.

Tourangeau, R. (2000). Remembering what happened: Memory errors and survey reports. In A. A. Stone, J. S. Turkkan, C. A. Bachrach, J. B. Jobe, H. S. Kurtzman & V. S. Cain (Eds.), *The science of self-report: Implications for research and practice* (pp. 29–47). Mahwah, NJ: Lawrence Erlbaum Associates.

Tucker, C. M., Fennell, R. S., Pedersen, T., Higley, B. P., Wallack, C. E., & Peterson, S. (2002). Associations with medication adherence among ethnically different pediatric patients with renal transplants. *Pediatric Nephrology, 17*, 251–256.

Tucker, C. M., Petersen, S., Herman, K. C., Fennell, R. S., Bowling, B., Pedersen, T., et al. (2001). Self-regulation predictors of medication adherence among ethnically different pediatric patients with renal transplants. *Journal of Pediatric Psychology, 26*, 455–464.

Urquhart, J. (1989). Noncompliance: The ultimate absorption barrier. In L. F. Prescott & W. S. Mimmo (Eds.), *Novel drug delivery and its therapeutic application* (pp. 127–137). New York: John Wiley & Sons.

Urquhart, J. (1994). Role of patient compliance in clinical pharmacokinetics: A review of recent research. *Clinical Pharmacokinetics, 27*, 202–215.

Urquhart, J., & De Klerk, E. (1998). Contending paradigms for the interpretation of data on patient compliance with therapeutic drug regimens. *Statistics in Medicine, 17*, 251–267.

Vandereycken, W., & Meermann, R. (1988). Chronic illness behavior and noncompliance with treatments: Pathways to an interactional approach. *Psychotherapy Psychosomatics, 50*, 182–191.

Van Dyke, R. B., Lee, S., Johnson, G. M., Wiznia, A., Mohan, K., Stanley, K., et al., (2002). Reported adherence as a determinant of response to highly active antiretroviral therapy in children who have human immunodeficiency virus infection. *Pediatrics, 109*, 1–7.

van Es, S. M., le Coq, E. M., Brouwer, A. I., Mesters, I., Nagelkerke, A. F., & Colland, V. T. (1998). Adherence-related behavior in adolescents with asthma: Results from focus group interviews. *Journal of Asthma, 35*, 637–646.

van Es, S. M., Nagelkerke, A. F., Colland, V. T., Scholten, R. J., & Bouter, L. M. (2001). A intervention programme using the ASE-model aimed at enhancing adherence in adolescents with asthma. *Patient Education and Counseling, 44*, 193–203.

Varni, J. W., Seid, M., & Rode, C. A.. (1999). The PedsQL: Measurement model for the pediatric quality of life inventory. *Medical Care, 37*, 126–139.

Varni, J. W., & Wallander, J. L. (1984). Adherence to health-related regimens in pediatric chronic disorders. *Clinical Psychology Review, 4*, 585–596.

Vrijens, B., & Goetghebeur, E. (1999). The impact of compliance on pharmacokinetic studies. *Statistical Methods in Medical Research, 8*, 247–262.

Walders, N., Kopel, S. J., Koins-Mitchell, D., & McQuaid, E. L. (2005). Patterns of quick-relief and long-term controller medication use in pediatric asthma. *Journal of Pediatrics, 146*, 177–182.

Walker, L. S., Garber, J., & Van Slyke, D. A. (1995). Do parents excuse the misbehavior of children with physical or emotional symptoms? An investigation of the pediatric sick role. *Journal of Pediatric Psychology, 20*, 329–345.

Webb, T. L., & Sheeran, P. (2006). Does changing behavioral intentions engender behavior change? A meta-analysis of the experimental evidence. *Psychological Bulletin, 132*, 249–268.

Wells, J. A., & Strickland, D. E. (1982). Physiogenic bias as invalidity in psychiatric symptom scales. *Journal of Health & Social Behavior, 23*, 235–252.

Westman, E., Ambler, G. R., Royle, M., Peat, J., & Chan, A. (1999). Children with coeliac disease and insulin dependent diabetes mellitus-growth, diabetes control and dietary intake. *Journal of Pediatric Endocrinology and Metabolism, 12*, 433–442.

Wicker, A. W. (1985). Getting out of our conceptual ruts: Strategies for expanding conceptual frameworks. *American Psychologist, 40*, 1094–1103.

Wiebe, D. J., Berg, C. A., Korbel, C., Palmer, D. L., Beveridge, R. M., Upchurch, R., et al., (2005). Children's appraisals of maternal involvement in coping with diabetes: Enhancing our understanding of adherence, metabolic control, and quality of life across adolescence. *Journal of Pediatric Psychology, 30*, 167–178.

Wiener, L., Riekert, K., Ryder, C., & Wood, L. V. (2004). Assessing medication adherence in adolescents with HIV when electronic monitoring is not feasible. *AIDS Patient Care and STDS, 18*, 527–538.

Wildman, B. G., & Erickson, M. T. (1977). Methodological problems in behavioral observation. In J. D. Cone & R. P. Hawkins (Eds.), *Behavioral assessment: New directions in clinical psychology* (pp. 255–273). New York: Brunner/Mazel.

Williams, P. L., Storm, D., Montepiedra, G., Nichols, S., Kammerer, B., Sirois, P. A., et al., (2006). Predictors of adherence to antiretroviral medications in children and adolescents with HIV infection. *Pediatrics, 118*, 1745–1757.

Williams, R., Maiman, L. A., Broadbent, D. M., Kotok, D., Lawrence, R. A., Longfield, L. A. et al., (1986). Educational strategies to improve compliance with an antibiotic regimen. *American Journal of Diseases of Children, 140*, 216–220.

Wilson, D. P., & Endres, R. K. (1986). Compliance with blood glucose monitoring in children with type I diabetes mellitus. *The Journal of Pediatrics, 108*, 1022–1024.

Wilson, K. G., Hayes, S. C., & Gifford, E. V. (1997). Cognition in behavior therapy: Agreements and differences. *Journal of Behavior Therapy & Experimental Psychiatry, 28*, 53–63.

Wing, R. R., Koeske, R., New, A., Lamparski, D., & Becker, D. (1986). Behavioral skills in self-monitoring of blood glucose: Relationship to accuracy. *Diabetes Care, 9*, 330–333.

Wing, R. R., Lamparski, D. M., Zaslow, S., Betschart, J., Simmens, L., & Becker, D. (1985). Frequency and accuracy of self-monitoring of blood glucose in children: Relationship to glycemic control. *Diabetes Care, 8*, 214–218.

Winnick, S., Lucas, D. O., Hartman, A. L., & Toll, D. (2005). How do you improve compliance? *Pediatrics, 115*, e718–e724.

Winter, M. E. (2003). *Basic clinical pharmacokinetics* (4th ed.). Hagerstown, MD: Lippincott Williams & Wilkins.

Wood, P. R., Casey, R., Kolski, G. B., & McCormick, M. C. (1985). Compliance with oral theophylline therapy in asthmatic children. *Annals of Allergy, 54*, 400–404.

World Health Organization (2003). *Adherence to long-term therapies: Evidence for action.* Geneva: Author.

Wu, Y. P., & Roberts, M. C. (2008). A meta-analysis of interventions to increase adherence to medications regimens for pediatric otitis media and streptococcal pharyngitis. *Journal of Pediatric Psychology, 33*, 789–796.

Wynn, K. S., & Eckel, E. M. (1986). Juvenile rheumatoid arthritis and home physical therapy program compliance. *Physical & Occupational Therapy in Pediatrics, 6*, 55–63.

Wysocki, T., & Gavin, L. (2006). Paternal involvement in the management of pediatric chronic diseases: Associations with adherence, quality of life, and health status. *Journal of Pediatric Psychology, 31*, 501–511.

Wysocki, T., Green, L., & Huxtable, K. (1989). Blood glucose monitoring by diabetic adolescents: Compliance and metabolic control. *Health Psychology, 8*, 267–284.

Wysocki, T., Harris, M. A., Buckloh, L. M., Mertlich, D., Lochrie, A. S., Taylor, A., et al., (2006). Effects of behavioral family systems therapy for diabetes on adolescents' family relationships, treatment adherence, and metabolic control. *Journal of Pediatric Psychology, 31*, 928–938.

Wysocki, T., Harris, M. A., Greco, P., Bubb, J., Danda, C. E., Harvey, L. M., et al., (2000). Randomized, controlled trial of behavior therapy for adolescents with insulin-dependent diabetes. *Journal of Pediatric Psychology, 25*, 23–33.

Yachha, S. K., Srivastava, A., Mohindra, S., Krishnani, N., & Aggarwal, R. (2007). Effect of a gluten-free diet on growth and small-bowel histology in children with celiac disease in India. *Journal of Gastroenterology and Hepatology, 22*, 1300–1305.

Yoman, J. (2008). A primer on functional analysis. *Cognitive & Behavioral Practice, 15*, 325–340.

Zifferblatt, S. M. (1975). Increasing patient compliance through the applied analysis of behavior. *Preventive Medicine, 4*, 173–182.

Zora, J. A., Lutz, C. N., & Tinkelman, D. G. (1989). Assessment of compliance in children using inhaled beta adrenergic agonists. *Annals of Allergy, 62*, 406–409.

Index

Note: The letters f and t following the locators refer to figures and tables respectively

A

Aaronson, N. K., 107, 112
Abadom, V., 23
ABA theory, *see* Applied behavior analytic
    (ABA) theory
Abetz, L., 30, 107
Abrams, E. J., 24, 25
Abshire, D. A., 153
Achenbach, T. M., 108, 110
Ackerson, L., 95
Ackloo, E., 152
Acute disease regimens
    adherence rates
        assessment criteria, example, 4
        in pediatrics, 5t–6t
        urine assays/pill counts, assessment
            to, 4
    in pediatrics, adherence intervention
        studies, 148t–150t
Acute pediatric diseases, 147–151,
    148t–150t, 177
Adams, C. D., 2, 3
Adesman, A. R., 39
Adherence
    definitions, 1–2
        by Haynes, 1
        by WHO, 2
    elements of
        behavior/advice, concordance, 2
        behavioral requirements, 1
        'extent,' 2
        health-care providers, role, 2
    importance of, 184–185
    intervention studies
        acute pediatric diseases, 147–151
    problems, types, 3–4
        drug holidays, consequences, 3
        nonadherence, unintentional/
            volitional, 3

rebound effect, drug toxicity, 3
rates
    acute disease regimens, 4–7
    chronic disease regimens, 7
"Adherence main effect," 36
Adherence measures, comparative performance
    electronic monitors/other measures
        of adherence in pediatric medicine,
        95t–101t
Adlis, S. A., 9
Aggarwal, R., 24
"Agreed recommendations," 2
Aiken, L. S., 36
Aims, assessment of adherence
    evaluation of intervention efforts, 71
    intervention selection
        nature of adherence problems, 70–71
        types of adherence problems,
            examples, 70
    prediction, 70
    screening and diagnosis, 69–70
Aitchison, T. C., 98
Ajzen, I., 55, 56, 57
Akçay, F., 20, 24
Albin, R. W., 142
Alekseev, L., 26
Algina, J., 103
Aligne, C. A., 118, 119
Allen, K. D., 142
Allergens, 50
Altemeier, W. A., 149
Altinkaynak, S., 24
Ambler, G. R., 24
Anand, V. K., 23
Anderson, B., 13
Anderson, B. J., 37, 40
Anderson, C. M., 37, 66
Anderson, H. A., 34
Anson, O., 19

Anti-inflammatory medication, 34, 50, 141
   nonsteroidal, 129
   oral, Naproxen, 66
Antiretroviral medications, 2, 112, 139, 181
Applied behavior analytic (ABA) theory,
      63–67
   appraisal
      "cognitivist challenge" to ABA
         model, 65
   clinical implications
      polyarticular JRA, strategies
         to adherence, 66–67
      14-year-old male with polyarticular
         JRA, example, 66
   contingency-shaped and rule-governed
      behavior, 63
   operant theory, effects on behavior,
      63, 64 f
   description, 63–64
      functional analysis, critical dimension
         of, 64
April, K. T., 26, 41
Apter, A. J., 94, 95
Arfken, C., 92
Arfken, C. L., 17
Aronson, N., 106
Asthma
   mortality, effect of nonadherence, 34
   patients, requirements
      inhaled anti-inflammatory
         medication, 50
      inhaled bronchodilator medication, 50
Athreya, B. H., 41, 107
"Attitudinal" theories, 57
Auslander, W. F., 37
Averbuch, M., 82
Avruskin, T. W., 37

B
Backes, J. M., 76
Baer, D. M., 63
Baker, S. A., 28
Baldassano, R. N., 21
Balson, P. M., 152
Balu, S., 35
Bandura, A., 48, 51, 52, 53, 54, 61, 65, 66
Bandura's concept of self-efficacy, 48
Barabino, A., 19
Barakat, L. P., 29, 41
Barlow, D. H., 180, 183, 184
Barnard, M. U., 4, 35, 41, 65, 77, 102, 122, 140
Barrios, B. A., 69, 71, 103, 104
Barron, A., 42

Bartholomew, L. K., 158
Bartlett, S. J., 8, 39
Bass, J. W., 148
Bauman, L. J., 8, 34, 139
Baum, D., 153
Bazzigaluppi, E., 20
Beck, D. E., 29, 37, 38, 40, 172
Becker, M. H., 19, 48, 50, 53, 149
Beck, S., 77
Behavioral checklists, purpose of, 77
Behavioral intentions, factors, 56 f
   attitude towards behavior, 56
   perceived behavioral control, 56
   subjective norms, 56
Behavioral strategies for improving adherence,
      127–140
   adherence incentives, 129–134
      negotiating and contracting for behavior
         change, 134 f
      token-system program, 130 f–131 f
   discipline strategies, 135–137
      skilled or effective discipline, 135
      time-out handout, 135 f–137 f
   parental monitoring and supervision,
      127–129
      parents of teenagers, 128
      regimen-monitoring form, 128 f
   prompting adherence, 129
      Hand-held PDA programs, 129
   psychotherapeutic interventions, 138
   self-management strategies, 138
      cognitive and contemporary
         behavior, 138
      problem-solving skills, 138
      psychotherapeutic interventions, 138
      treatments/diseases with positive/
         negative consequences, 139t
   See also Improvement strategies
         of adherence
Belëndez, M., 165
Bellack, A. S., 79
Bell-Dolan, D. J., 79
Bell, G. L., 90
Belmont, J. M., 8, 9, 28, 182
Bender, B., 95
Bender, B. G., 8, 41
Benet, L. Z., 74
Berg, C. J., 8, 9
Berg, J. S., 35, 39
Bergman, A. B., 5, 7
Berkovitch, M., 82, 176
Berrien, V. M., 170
Bertakis, K. D., 148

Blackmore, A. M., 159
Blaschke, T., 2
Blaschke, T. F., 104
Bloom, B. R., 34
Blount, R. L., 50
Blowey, D. L., 30, 79, 96
Blue, J. W., 106
Blumenstock, G., 4
Bobrow, E. S., 37, 39, 40, 42, 49
Boccuti, L., 77
Boggs, S. R., 107, 172
Bohane, T. D., 23
Bollinger, M. E., 96
Bond, G. G., 36, 37, 40, 42, 49, 89
Bond, W. S., 84, 92, 102
Bonner, S., 153
Borch, R. F., 76
Boréus, L. O., 77
Bouter, L. M., 153
Bovaird, J. A., 30
Boyer, A., 177
Brackett, J., 13
Brackis-Cott, E., 24, 25
Braes, P. U., 157
Bransford, J. D., 85
Branstetter, A. D., 9, 39, 53
Brazeau, M., 6
Breese, B. B., 5
Brewer, E. J., 26, 42
Brink, S., 53
Bronchodilator medication, 50, 51, 54, 134
Brooks, A. J., 40, 41, 42
Brooks-Gunn, J., 76
Brownbridge, G., 37, 39, 40, 41
Brownlee-Duffeck, M., 50, 89
Brown, S. J., 143, 161
Burge, D. A., 79
Burkhart, P. V., 153
Burroughs, T. E., 40
Bursch, B., 50
Bush, P. J., 48, 49
Buston, K. M., 42
Butz, A. M., 96
Buu, A., 107

C
Cadman, D., 108
Cairns, G. F., 11
Cairns, N. U., 11
Cameron, J., 11
Cantrill, J. A., 143
Carlino, P., 147, 149
Carlsen, K.-H., 7

Carney, R. M., 161
Carroll, M. S., 151
Carton, J. S., 172
Cary, J., 76
Casey, R., 10, 148
Catania, A. C., 53
Catto-Smith, A. G., 23
CD-ROM or web-based program for enhancing
    adherence, elements of, 143–145,
    144t
Celano, M., 9, 40, 42, 77
Chan, A., 24
Chan, D. S., 145, 154
Channell, S., 90
Charney, E., 5
Chasalow, F., 10
CHBM, see The Children's Health Belief
    Model (CHBM)
Cheang, M. S., 10
Chemlik, F., 97
Chesney, M. A., 36
The Children's Health Belief Model (CHBM),
    48, 49f
    caretaker, role of, 48, 49f
    study, factors used/limitations, 49
Christensen, N. K., 15
Christophersen, E. R., 27, 36, 69, 73, 84,
    119, 149
Chronic disease regimens, 4, 7, 43, 61, 71, 102,
    119, 121, 123, 130, 140, 151
    adherence rates in pediatrics, 8t–31t
    HIV/GI disorders, study, 7
    medication/non-medication regimens,
        adherence rates, 7
Chronic pediatric diseases, 151–152,
    153t–176t
    insulin-dependent diabetes children's
        regimen, 151–152
Chudziker, G. M., 5
Cipani, E., 135
Clark, N. M., 48, 57, 181
Cleemput, I., 35
Clinical implications of correlates, 43–45
    disease-related correlates, 44
    parental monitoring, importance, 43
    patient/family correlates, 43–44
    regimen-related correlates, 44–45
    static/immutable variables, examples, 43
Clinically significant nonadherence
    (CSN), 183
Cluss, P. A., 9, 34, 76
Cobden, D., 35
Cognitive/self-mediated thought processes, 67

Cohen, J., 152
Cohen, L. L., 93, 108
Cohen, M., 149
Cohen, N., 165
Colburn, W. A., 106
Colcher, I. S., 148
Coleman, J. C., 50
Colland, V. T., 157
Competent functioning, 52
Contingency-shaped and rule-governed
        behavior, *see* Applied behavior
        analytic (ABA) theory
Contingency-shaped behavior
    operant processes, effects on behavior
        negative punishment/reinforcement, 63
        positive punishment/reinforcement, 63
Controlled clinical trials (RCTs), 183
Corcoran, K. J., 54
Correlates of adherence
    cautions
        causal relationship development,
            conditions, 42
    clinical implications, 43–45
        disease-related correlates, 44
        parental monitoring, importance, 43
        patient/family correlates, 43–44
        regimen-related correlates, 44–45
        static/immutable variables,
            examples, 43
    disease-related correlates, 40–41
        course, 40
        duration, 40
        perceived severity, 41
        symptoms/disease severity, 40–41
    nonadherence risk profile, 42–43
    patient/family correlates, 37–40
        barriers, 40
        demographics, 37
        family adjustment and coping, 39–40
        knowledge, 38
        parental involvement/monitoring, 40
        patient adjustment and coping, 38–39
        patient gender, correlate
            of adherence, 37
        race, 38
        SES and family composition, 37–38
    reasons for examining, 36–37
    regimen-related correlates, 41–42
        costs, 41
        efficacy, 42
        side effects, 41–42
        type and complexity, 41
Coutts, J. A. P., 9, 79

Cox, C., 82
Cramer, J. A., 79, 82
Crandall, W. V., 22
Creer, T. L., 153
Crocker, L., 103
Croft, D. R., 119
"Cross-informant variance," 108
CSN, *see* Clinically significant nonadherence
        (CSN)
Cuffari, C., 20, 23
"Culturally sensitive model," 38
Cummings, K. M., 40
Cunningham, P. B., 171
Cuskey, W. R., 27, 37, 40
Cystic fibrosis (CF)
    application of SCT to, 54–55
    medical regimen of 7-year-old female
        with, 54
Czajkowski, D. R., 12
Czajkowski, S. M., 36

D
Da Costa, I. G., 130, 154
Dahlström, B., 86
Dahms, W. T., 134
Daily Count Index (DCI), 104
Daschner, F., 5
Data interpretation, adherence measurement
    units of analysis/formulas
        Daily Count Index (DCI), 104
        Exact Daily Adherence (EAC), 105
        Fraction of Doses (Fr), 104
        Prescribed Intervals Method (PI), 105
        Therapeutic Coverage (TC), 105
Davies, P., 23
Davies, W. H., 166
Davis, C. L., 89
Davis, C. M., 21
Davis, M. A., 143
Davis, T., 161
Dawes, R. M., 85
Dawson, K. P., 176
Day, A. S., 23
DCI, *see* Daily Count Index (DCI)
Deaton, A. V., 3
Deci, E. L., 65
Decisional balance, meaning, 59
DeCuir-Whalley, S., 11
DeGeest, S., 35
Delamater, A. M., 17, 89
DeLambo, K. E., 88
De la Sota, A., 156
Dell, R., 76

Demir, H., 20
Denson-Lino, J. M., 37
DeVellis, B. M., 52, 53
DeVellis, R. F., 52
Devries, J. M., 94
Diabetes, Type 1, 61–62
    medical regimen of 16-year-old male with,
        61–62
        application of TTM to, 62
The Diagnostic and Statistical Manual of
        Mental Disorders (DSM-IV), 70
Dickey, F. F., 5
DiClemente, C. C., 58, 61
DiMatteo, M. R., 105
Dinakar, C., 2
Dischler, J., 35
Discipline strategies, 135–137
    skilled or effective discipline, 135
    time-out handout, 136 f–137 f
    See also Improvement strategies
        of adherence
Disease and adherence/health outcomes
        assessment
    adherence assessment, aim
        intervention efforts, evaluation of, 71
        intervention selection, 70–71
        prediction, 70
        screening and diagnosis, 69–70
    adherence measurement,
            issues/recommendations
        clinical and treatment utility, 105–106
        clinicians and researchers, role of, 102,
            103, 104
        data interpretation, 104–105
        directness, 103
        measurement standards, 103–104
        reactivity, 102
        representativeness, 102–103
    assessment strategies, assets/liabilities
        adherence measures, comparative
            performance, 94–102
        assets/liabilities of adherence
            measures, 74t
        drug assays, 74–77
        electronic monitors, 79–83
        observation, 77–79
        patient/parental reports, 86–94
        pill counts, 83–84
        provider estimates, 84–85
    disease/health measures,
            issues/recommendations
        choice of informants, 108

generic vs. disease-specific
        measures, 109
    psychometric standards,
        see Psychometric standards
        of adherence
    representativeness, 108–109
    disease/health outcomes assessment,
        106–107
    patients, assessment
        adherence monitoring, informants/
            assessors role, 73
        patient/parent regimen-related
            behaviors, 73
        training/quality control progams
            to informants, 73
    target behaviors
        guidelines for selection, see Target
            behaviors for assessing adherence,
            selection of
Disease-related correlates, 40–41
    course, 40
    duration, 40
    perceived severity, 41
    symptoms/disease severity, 40–41
Disney, F. A., 5
Doershuk, C. F., 135
Dohil, R., 20
Dolezal, C., 24, 25
Donithan, M., 96
Doughty, A., 97
Downs, J. A., 159
Drabman, R. S., 160
Dracup, K. A., 2
Dreyer, M. L., 2, 30
Drotar, D., 11, 16, 39, 73, 88, 111, 135, 139,
        143, 145, 177
Drug assays
    absorption of drugs
        oral administration of drugs, effects,
            74–75
    assets/liabilities, 76–77
    bioavailability of drug, factors affecting, 75
    drug metabolism
        enzymatic reactions, result of, 75
        liver enzymes, role in, 75
    elimination/excretion of drug
        by urination, 75
"Drug holiday," 3
Drug-resistant microbes, 34
Drug(s)
    absorption, 74–75
    bioavailability of
        half-life, 75

Drug(s) (*cont.*)
    steady state, 75
    elimination/excretion
      by urination, 75
    metabolism
      enzymatic reactions, result of, 75
    plasma level, 3
DSM-IV, *see* The Diagnostic and Statistical
    Manual of Mental Disorders
    (DSM-IV)
D statistics, 152
    See also Meta-analytic reviews
      of adherence interventions
Duffy, C. M., 26
Dulberg, C., 5
Dunbar-Jacob, J. M., 153
Dunbar, J. M., 115

E
Eckel, E. M., 39
Eckernäs, S. A., 86
Educational strategies for improving
    adherence, 116–121
    content and objectives of education,
      116–117
      benefits of consistent adherence and
        strategies, 117
      information needs about the disease,
        116–117
      negative side effects of treatment, 117
    factors to consider when developing health
      education materials, 119*t*
    goals of education
      knowing that and *knowing how*
      (Ryle), 116
      reference of patients with diabetes, 116
    strategies, 117–120
      handouts by drug companies, 119, 120 *f*
      instructions for using a metered-dose
        inhaler, 120 *f*
      modeling and behavioral rehearsal,
        120 *f*
      ongoing process, 117
      pamphlets and information on Web
        sites, 118
      verbal communication, 117–118
      written communication and other
        media, 118–119
Edwards, T. C., 107
Effect size (ES) estimate, 152
    See also Meta-analytic reviews
      of adherence interventions
Eggleston, P. A., 185

Eidson, M., 17
Eisenberger, R., 65
Eiser, C., 107
Eisler, I., 31
El-Charr, G. M., 42
Electronic monitors
    application of, 79
    assets/liabilities, 80–83
    See also Medication Event Monitoring
      System (MEMS®)
Ellis, D. A., 40, 44, 161, 162
Ellison, R. S., 149
Enactive mastery, 55
Endres, R. K., 18
Eney, R. D., 9, 151, 154
Enhancement factors for self-efficacy
    enactive mastery, 55
    verbal persuasion, 55
    vicarious experiences, 55
Epstein, L. H., 9, 34, 36, 76, 77, 151, 163
Epstein, R. S., 35
Erickson, M. T., 78, 79, 102
Ertekin, V., 20, 24
Espelage, D. L., 73, 88
Ettenger, R. B., 30, 33
Evers, K. E., 59
Exact Daily Adherence (EAC), 105

F
Faier-Routman, J., 111
Farkas, G. M., 77
Farley, J., 90, 98
Farley, J. J., 25
Farmer, K. C., 73
Faust, D., 85
Feinstein, A. R., 112
Feinstein, S., 30, 37, 40
Feldman, D. E., 26, 34, 37, 41
Feldman, H. I., 94
Feldman, W., 5
Fennell, R. S., 172
Ferguson, A. E., 98
Ferrus, S., 90
Festa, R. S., 10, 39
Fielding, D. M., 37, 39, 40, 41
Figueroa, J., 77
Fink, D., 149
Finkelstein, D., 13
Finley, R., 177
Finney, J. W., 69, 84, 149
Fireman, P., 9, 34, 153
Fishbein, M., 55
Fisher, C. B., 143

Fivush, B. A., 30
Fletcher, R. H., 36, 110
Fletcher, S. W., 36
Flowers, N. T., 104
Fobil, J. N., 143
Follansbee, D., 37
Forbes, G. B., 76
Forbis, S., 118, 119
Forster, D., 143
Foster, S. L., 79
Foulkes, L. M., 172
Foye, H. R., 76
Fraction of Doses (Fr), 104
Francis, A. B., 5
Frazier, T., 177
Fredericks, E. M., 34
Freund, A., 37, 86
Frey, M., 44
Friday, G., 9, 34
Fried, A. L., 143
Friedman, I. M., 28, 38, 39
Fries, J. F., 107
Friman, P. C., 69, 71, 78, 142, 149
Fritz, G. K., 9
Fuchs, R., 53
Furth, S. L., 30

G
Galvis, S. A., 9, 34
Garber, J., 135
Garvie, P. A., 125, 171
Gastrointestinal (GI) disorders, 7
Gavin, L., 39, 151, 152
Gavin, L. A., 92
Geffken, G., 145
Geiss, S. K., 39
Gelfand, K., 145
Geller, R. J., 9, 77
Generic *vs.* disease-specific measures, 109
Gerber, M. A., 5
Gerich, J., 118
Gerson, A. C., 30, 39, 79
Gerstner, T. V., 10
Giannini, E. H., 26, 42
Gibbons, A., 34, 35
Gibson, N. A., 9, 98
GI disorders, *see* Gastrointestinal (GI)
        disorders
Gifford, E. V., 66
Gilbert, A., 169
Gilbert, B. O., 77
Gilbert, D. T., 85
Gilbert, J., 50

Gill, N., 112
Gill, T. M., 112
Ginsburg, C. M., 5
Glasgow, R. E., 39, 41, 49, 50, 166
Glauser, T. A., 3
Glazebrook, C., 143
Glowasky, A., 148
Goetghebeur, E., 36
Golden, M. P., 40
Goldring, J. M., 34
Goldsmith, D. P., 107
Goldstein, A., 6
Goldstein, D., 89
Goldstein, E. O., 9, 151, 154
Goldstein, G. L., 130
Goldsten, D., 7
Goodwin, D. A. J., 107
Gordis, L., 4, 6, 86, 94, 105, 112, 158
Graber, J. A., 76
Graham-Pole, J., 107
Graves, M. M., 177, 178, 179, 180
Gray, N. J., 143
Greco, P., 89
Greenan-Fowler, E., 170
Greenberg, M., 11
Green, B. F., 107
Greening, L., 13, 39
Green, J. L., 5
Green, L., 167
Greycloud, M. A., 149
Groopman, J., 85
Gross, A. M., 151, 163
Grossman, H. Y., 53
Grotz, W., 4
Grum, C. M., 181
Gudas, L. J., 36, 37, 38, 39, 41, 49, 84
Guerin, B., 50, 57
Guevara, J. P., 181

H
Hagopian, L. P., 159
Hains, A. A., 166
'Half-life' of drug, definition, 75
Halsey-Lyda, M., 145
Halterman, J. S., 185
Hammersley-Maercklein, G., 39
Hansen, C. A., 37
Harmon, W. E., 39
Harris, C. V., 106, 107, 110
Harris, M., 92
Hartman, A. L., 125
Hartman, C., 21
Haskard, K. B., 105

Hassall, E., 20
Hauser, S. T., 39, 53
Havermans, G., 53
Hawkins, R. M. F., 53
Hawkins, R. P., 66
Hayes, S. C., 53, 54, 63, 64, 105, 138
Hayford, J. R., 27, 41
Haynes, R. B., 1, 2, 152, 181
Haynes, S. M., 42
Haynes, S. N., 64, 142
Hazzard, A., 28, 39, 41
HBM, see Health belief model (HBM)
Health belief model (HBM), 48–51
    appraisal, 48–50
        conceptual/methodological grounds,
            criticism on, 49–50
        pediatric medical adherence, 49
    clinical implications, 50–51
        asthma, strategies to adherence, 50–51
        See also Behavioral intentions, factors
    description, 48
    variables
        cues to action, 48
        perceived barriers/benefits, 48
        perceived severity/susceptibility, 48
    See also The Children's Health Belief
        Model (CHBM)
Health outcomes and adherence assessment,
        measurement issues
    assessment, aims
        intervention efforts, evaluation
            of, 71
        intervention selection, 70–71
        prediction, 70
        screening and diagnosis, 69–70
    assessment strategies, assets/liabilities
        adherence measures, comparative
            performance, 94–102
        assets/liabilities of adherence
            measures, 74t
        drug assays, 74–77
        electronic monitors, 79–83
        observation, 77–79
        patient/parental reports, 86–94
        pill counts, 83–84
        provider estimates, 84–85
    disease/health measures,
            issues/recommendations
        choice of informants, 108
        generic vs. disease-specific
            measures, 109

psychometric standards,
    see Psychometric standards
    of adherence
    representativeness, 108–109
disease/health outcomes assessment,
    106–107
measurement, issues/recommendations
    clinical and treatment utility, 105–106
    clinicians and researchers, role of, 102,
        103, 104
    data interpretation, 104–105
    directness, 103
    measurement standards, 103–104
    reactivity, 102
    representativeness, 102–103
patients, assessment of
    adherence monitoring, informants/
        assessors role, 73
    patient/parent regimen-related
        behaviors, 73
    training/quality control progams
        to informants, 73
target behaviors
    guidelines for selection, see Target
        behaviors for assessing adherence,
        selection of
Health-related quality of life (HRQOL), 106
    core domains of, 107
Heath, K. V., 3
Heidgerken, A. D., 145
Hein, K., 76
Heisenberg Uncertainty Principle, 104
Heisenberg, W., 104
Hemoglobin A1C, 107
Hendeles, L., 94
Hendry, L., 50
Henley, M., 39
Henness, D. M., 6
Hentinen, M., 13
Hermann, C., 79
Herrold, A. J., 40
Hersen, M., 79, 180
Hinds, P. S., 90
Hines, S., 90
HIV, see Human immunodeficiency virus
    (HIV)
Hobbs, S. A., 12, 39
Hobson, D., 17
Hoekelman, R. A., 94
Hogg, R. S., 3
Ho, J., 13
Holmbeck, G. N., 90
Holmes, C. S., 37, 38, 39, 40

Hommel, K. A., 21
Hommell, K. A., 145
Hook, R. J., 69
Hoppe, J. E., 4, 6
Horner, R. H., 64, 142
Horwitz, R. I., 36
Horwitz, S. M., 36
Houle, C. R., 48, 57
Hovell, 115
Howe, C. J., 164
Howell, C. T., 108
Howe, S., 107
HRQOL, *see* Health-related quality of life
        (HRQOL)
Human immunodeficiency virus (HIV)
    antiretroviral medications, 2
    lower adherence to antiretroviral
        drugs, 34
Hussar, D. A., 84, 92, 102
Hutchinson, S. J., 28
Huxtable, K., 167

I
Iannotti, R. J., 14, 48, 49
Ievers, C. E., 135
Ievers-Landis, C. E., 7, 73, 88
Improvement strategies of adherence
    behavioral strategies, 127–140
    educational strategies, 116–121
    individualizing interventions
        barriers adherence interview answer
            choices, 141 *f*
        barriers to adherence, 140–141
        functional analysis, 142–143
    organizational strategies, 121–127
    technology-based interventions, 143–145
Incentives, 129–134
    negotiating and contracting for behavior
        change, 134 *f*
    token-system program, 130 *f*–131 *f*
    See also Improvement strategies of
        adherence
Ingersoll, G. M., 40
Insulin-dependent diabetes children's regimen,
        151–152
Interventions
    barriers, mentioned by JRA patient, 141
    barriers to adherence, 140–141
    CD-ROM or Web-based interventions, 143,
        144–145, 144 *f*
    functional analysis, 142–143
        steps for conducting, 142–143
    individualizing

barriers adherence interview answer
    choices, 141 *f*
barriers to adherence, 140–141
functional analysis, 142–143
    See also Interventions
nature of adherence problems
    clinicians, role of, 71
    patients who overdose, 70
    patients who underdose, 70
technology-based, 143–145
    barriers to be addressed, 143
    CD-ROM or Web-based
        interventions, 143
telehealth, 145
Intervention studies on improving adherence
        to regimens
    acute pediatric diseases, 147–151,
        148 *f*–150 *f*
    chronic pediatric diseases, 151–152,
        153 *t*–176 *t*
        insulin-dependent diabetes children's
            regimen, 151–152
    importance of adherence, 184–185
    meta-analytic reviews
        acute pediatric diseases, 177
        for adults, 152–177
        chronic pediatric diseases, 177–180
        conclusions from, 180–181
    studies targeting acute disease regimens
        in pediatrics, 148 *f*–150 *f*
    top tenways to advance research, 181–184
        See also Research on pediatric medical
            adherence, tenways to advance
Israel, D. M., 20
Iyengar, S., 7

J
Jacobson, A. M., 7, 14, 15, 37, 38, 39, 40
James, C., 143
James, D. S., 34
Jamieson, A., 176
Janz, N. K., 48, 50
Jarrett, R. B., 105
Jarzembowski, T., 33
Jenkins, S. C., 159
Jensen, S. A., 29, 38
Johanson, C. E., 74, 75, 77
Johnson, S., 58
Johnson, S. B., 37, 72, 77, 86, 93, 94, 102,
        106, 107
Johnson, T., 22, 23
Johnston, J. M., 47, 69, 73, 77, 102, 103
Jónasson, G., 7, 9, 37

Jordan, S. S., 13
Joshi, A. V., 35
Journal of Applied Behavior Analysis, 65, 142
JRA, *see* Juvenile rheumatoid arthritis (JRA)
Judd, B. A., 94
Jue, S. G., 82
Julius, S. M., 94, 99
Jung, D. C., 37
Juniper, E. F., 107
Juvenile idiopathic arthritis
    lower adherence to anti-inflammatory
        medications, 34
Juvenile rheumatoid arthritis (JRA), 38

K

Kahana, S., 177, 178
Kamps, J. L., 155, 183
Kanani, R., 152
Kaplan, M., 156
Kaplan, R. M., 92, 106
Kapur, G., 23
Kasprzyk, K. D., 55
Kastrissios, H., 104, 152, 181
Kavanagh, T., 112
Kazak, A. E., 43
Kazdin, A. E., 65, 66, 79
Kelloway, J. S., 9, 37
Kendall, P. C., 138
Kennard, B. D., 10, 39
Kessler, J. H., 160
Kesteloot, K., 35
"Keystone" behaviors, 72
Kidder, D. P., 129
Kirpalani, H., 108
Klein, J. D., 143
Klein, R. B., 9
Klemp, S., 89
Klinnert, M. D., 9, 87, 92
Klover, R. V., 17
Kniker, W. T., 155
Knowing that and *knowing how* (Ryle), 116
Kodish, E., 11
Koeske, R., 19
Kofi, O. A., 143
Kohlenberg, B. S., 64
Koins-Mitchell, D., 10
Kolaèek, S., 21
Kolski, G. B., 10
Konishi, C., 13
Koocher, G. P., 36
Kopel, S. J., 9, 10
Koren, G., 11, 79
Kovacs, M., 7, 15, 37, 39, 40

Kramer, J. C., 39
Krasner, L., 47
Kratochwill, T. R., 71
Krawiecki, N., 28
Krishnani, N., 24
Krishna, S., 143
Kruse, W., 79
Kuhn, T. S., 67
Kulik, J. A., 147, 149
Kumar, P. J., 21
Kumar, V. S., 164
Kurtin, P. S., 30, 39
Kuzmina, N., 26
Kvien, T. K., 27
Kyngas, H., 13

L

Labay, L., 50
Laffel, L., 13
Laffel, L. M., 164
Laffel, L. M. B., 164
La Greca, A. M., 37, 38, 39, 40, 43, 89, 151
Lamparski, D., 19
Lancaster, D., 11
Landgraf, J. M., 30, 107
Lansky, S. B., 11, 38
Lanzkowsky, P., 10
Lask, B., 31
Lau, R. C. W., 11, 79
Lavigne, J. V., 111
Lawson, M. L., 165
LeBaron, S., 155
Lee, D., 23
Lee, P., 58
Lee, W. C., 35
Lehane, E., 3
Lemanek, K., 130
Lennard, L., 11
Lensing, S., 125
Le Souëf, P. N., 159
Leventhal, J. M., 139
Lewandowski, A., 39
Lewis, C. E., 156
Lewis, M. A., 156
Ley, P., 157
Lilienfeld, A. M., 6
Lilleyman, J. S., 11
Lindsley, C. B., 27, 28, 64, 73
Lipsey, M. W., 152
Liptak, G. S., 147
Litt, I. F., 27, 37, 38, 40
Liver enzymes, 75
    structure/functioning, impact on drug
        metabolism, 75

Logan, D., 50
Lorenz, R. A., 15, 37, 77
Lovell, D. J., 42, 129
Lowe, K., 77, 165
Lowman, J. T., 11
Lucas, D. O., 125
Ludgwig, S., 148
Lutfey, K. E., 1
Lutz, C. N., 10
Lutzker, J. R., 77, 165

M

MacKenzie, R., 6
Mackner, L. M., 22, 160
Madigan, S., 89
Magalnick, L. J., 163
Magee, J. C., 33, 34
Magrab, P. R., 172
Mahoney, M. J., 65
Maikranz, J. M., 30, 79
Maiman, L. A., 76, 147, 149
Maisto, S. A., 85
Malasanos, T., 145
Mallon, J. C., 40
Malloy, M. J., 149
Malone, J., 37
Malone, P. S., 85
Mammography screening, 57
Mardy, G., 42
Marget, W., 5
Marhefka, S. L., 92
Mariani, P., 22
Marklein, J., 4
Markowitz, M., 6, 158
Marks, M. I., 6
Marosi, A., 156
Marshall, G. D., 115
Martin, F., 149
Martin, S., 25, 34
Mash, E. J., 69, 71, 77, 78, 79
Mason, B. J., 82
Matsui, D., 11, 42, 79
Matsuyama, J. R., 82
Mattar, M. E., 5
Mattar, M. F., 4, 6, 150
McCarthy, G., 3
McCarty, J. M., 4
McCaul, K. D., 39, 41, 42, 49, 166
McConaughy, S. H., 108
McCormick, M. C., 10, 41
McDonald, H. P., 177
McGrath, P. A., 108
McGuigan, K. A., 35

McKay, K., 170
McKeever, L. C., 150
McKibbon, K. A., 152
McLinn, S. E., 4, 6
McPherson, A. C., 143
McQuaid, E. L., 9, 10, 37, 38, 39, 43, 79, 87, 92
MDI, *see* Metered dose inhaler (MDI)
Meade, C. D., 118, 119
Measurement issues, adherence and health outcomes
  assessment of adherence
    intervention efforts, evaluation of, 71
    intervention selection, 70–71
    prediction, 70
    screening and diagnosis, 69–70
  assessment strategies, assets/liabilities
    adherence measures, comparative performance, 94–102
    assets/liabilities of adherence measures, 74*t*
    drug assays, 74–77
    electronic monitors, 79–83
    observation, 77–79
    patient/parental reports, 86–94
    pill counts, 83–84
    provider estimates, 84–85
  generic methodological issues/recommendations
    clinical and treatment utility, 105–106
    clinicians and researchers, role of, 102, 103, 104
    data interpretation, 104–105
    directness, 103
    measurement standards, 103–104
    reactivity, 102
    representativeness, 102–103
  health measures, issues/recommendations
    choice of informants, 108
    generic *vs.* disease-specific measures, 109
    psychometric standards, *see* Psychometric standards of adherence
    representativeness, 108–109
  health outcomes assessment, 106–107
  patients, assessment
    adherence monitoring, informants/ assessors role, 73
    patient/parent regimen-related behaviors, 73
    training/quality control progams to informants, 73

Measurement issues (*cont.*)
  target behaviors
    guidelines for selection, *see* Target
      behaviors for assessing adherence,
      selection of
Med, C., 4
Medical practice, culture of, 3
Medication Event Monitoring System
    (MEMS®)
  components of
    communicator module, 79
    monitor, 79
  example of data from, 81 *f*
Meehl, P. E., 85
Meermann, R., 3
Meichenbaum, D., 65
Melancon, S. M., 64
Meleis, A. I., 2
Mellins, C. A., 24, 25
Mellis, C. M., 157
Memory devices, 4
MEMS® SmartCap, 80
MEMS® TrackCap, 79
Méndez, F. J., 165
Messer, M. A., 107
Meta-analytic reviews of adherence
    interventions
  acute pediatric diseases, 177
  for adults, 152–177
  chronic pediatric diseases, 177–180
  conclusions from, 180–181
Metered dose inhaler (MDI), 77
  checklist, 78 *f*
Mikkelsen, T., 164
Milgrom, H., 95, 101
Miller, J. P., 37
Miller, S. T., 160
Miller, V. A., 16, 39
Millstein, S. G., 50
Mitchell, J. R., 74
Mitchell, W. G., 28
Model(s), *see individual*
Modi, A. C., 3, 7, 12, 28, 40, 50, 79, 87, 92,
    100, 107, 127, 140, 141, 145
Mohindra, S., 24
Moll, G., 13
Momy, J., 5
Montaner, J. S. G., 3
Montaño, D. E., 55, 57
Mora, S., 22
Morey, L., 85
Morita, D. A., 3
Morris, E. K., 65, 66

Morse, E. V., 152
Morse, R., 107
Mowinckel, P., 7
Muir, A., 145
Murphy, M. S., 22, 23
Murray, C. J. L., 34
Musk, A., 90
Myers, R. S., 61

N
Naar-King, S., 17, 37, 39, 44, 92, 171
Nagelkerke, A. F., 157
Naidoo, D., 23
Naproxen, 66
Narayan, S., 23
Nazarian, L. F., 147
Nelson, R. O., 105
Neu, A. M., 30
New, A., 19
Newacheck, P. W., 34
The "new gold standard," *see* Electronic
    monitors
Nightingale, E. O., 50
Nock, M. K., 180
Nonadherence
  consequences, 35–36
    active/placebo medications, adherence
      effects, 35–36
    "adherence main effect," 36
    clinical decisions, 35
  diagnosis of, 70
  health/well-being effects, 33–34
    African-American/Caucasian children,
      asthma-related death rates, 34
    anti-inflammatory medications, 34
    antiretroviral drugs, 34
    asthma in children/adolescents, 34
    immunosuppressive drugs, 33
    living/dead donor kidney
      transplantations, survival
      rates, 33
    microbial organisms, 'inoculation'
      of, 34
    tuberculosis reemergence, 34
  medical care, cost-effectiveness of, 34–35
    higher adherence, lower disease-related
      medical costs, 35
  pharmacokinetics, negative impact on, 36
  risk profile, 42–43
  unintentional, 3
    memory devices for patients with, 4
  volitional, 3
    medication side effects, 3

"Noncompliance with Treatment," code, 70
Nonsteroidal anti-inflammatory medications
            (NSAIDS), 80
Norcross, J. C., 58
Noyce, P. R., 143
NSAIDS, *see* Nonsteroidal anti-inflammatory
            medications (NSAIDS)

O

O Ailin, A., 199
Oakley, M. G., 153
O'Brien, W. H., 64, 141
Obrosky, D. S., 7
O'Callaghan, A., 23
O'Connor, R. D., 37
O'Donohue, W., 47
Oermann, M. H., 118, 119
Ohene-Frempong, K., 29
O'Leary, A., 52, 53
Oliva-Hemker, M. M., 23
Oliver, M. R., 23
Olivieri, N. F., 29, 79, 101
Olson, N. Y., 28
O'Neill, R. E., 142
Ooi, C. Y., 23
Opipari, L. C., 92, 160
Oral corticosteroids, 54
Oral pancreatic enzyme replacement, 54
Organizational strategies for improving
            adherence, 121–127
    consumer-friendly clinical settings,
            121–122
    increasing accessibility to health care, 121
        contact with social service
            agencies, 121
        outreach clinics, 121
    increasing provider supervision, 122–123,
            123 f–124 f
        clinic visits/follow-up, 122
        "report line" or phone number, 122
        written treatment plan, 123 f–124 f
    side effects of regimens
        minimize side effects, 125
    simplifying and minimizing negative side
            effects of regimens
        oral liquid medications, 125
        pill-swallowing protocol used for
            children with cystic fibrosis,
            126t–127t
        reducing complexity, 125
        tailoring regimens to patients'
            lifestyles/schedules, 125
    See also Improvement strategies of
            adherence

Orrbine, E., 165
Orr, D. P., 40
O'Shaughnessy, M. V., 3
Osterberg, L., 2
Ostosh, L., 118

P

Page, E. G., 151
Pai, A. L. H., 11
Palermo, T. M., 86, 107, 183
Palmer-Shevlin, N., 35
Parcel, G. S., 54
Parental monitoring and supervision, 127–129
    parents of teenagers, 128
    regimen-monitoring form, 128 f
Park, D. C., 129
Parker, C. C., 38
Parks, B. R., 38
Parton, E., 166
Pashos, C. L., 35
Passero, M. A., 13, 41
Patient/family correlates, 37–40
    adherence correlates to medical regimens,
            37–40
        barriers, 40
        demographics, 37
        family adjustment and coping, 39–40
        knowledge, 38
        parental involvement/monitoring, 40
        patient adjustment and coping, 38–39
        race, 38
        SES, 37–38
    barriers, 40
    demographics, 37
    family adjustment and coping, 39–40
    knowledge, 38
    parental involvement/monitoring, 40
    patient adjustment and coping, 38–39
    patient gender, correlate of adherence, 37
    race, 38
    SES and family composition, 37–38
Patient/parental reports
    assessment strategy, assets/liabilities,
            92–94
    daily diaries, 86
    global ratings, 86
    structured interviews and
            questionnaires, 86
        reliability/validity and self-report
            measures of adherence, 87t–91t
Patino, A. M., 17, 37, 38, 49
Paton, J. Y., 9, 98
Patrick, D. L., 107

Patterson, J. M., 37, 38, 39, 44, 125
Patwari, A. K., 23
Peat, J., 24
Pedan, A., 8
Pediatric medical adherence
    HBM rated by adults/adolescents
        asthma/cancer, better adherence, 49
        diabetes/cystic fibrosis, lower
            adherence, 49
    research, 181–184
        See also Research on pediatric medical
            adherence, ten ways to advance
Penkower, L., 31, 39
Pennypacker, H. S., 47, 69, 73, 77, 102, 103
Pentland, A., 164
Perceived barriers, definition, 48
Perceived behavioral control, 56, 57
Perceived benefits, definition, 48
Perceived self-efficacy, definition, 52
Perceived severity, definition, 48
Perceived susceptibility, definition, 48
Perrin, E. C., 111, 139
Perrotta, R., 4
Petersen, A. C., 50
Peterson, A. M., 177, 180
Peterson, L., 89
Peterson, M. W., 119
Phillips, K. M., 9, 77
Phipps, S., 11, 90
PI, *see* Prescribed Intervals Method (PI)
Piaget's theory, 60
Pichert, J. W., 15
Pichichero, M. E., 4, 6
Pieper, K. B., 64, 73, 83, 130, 173
Pill counts, 83–84
    assets/liabilities, 83–84
Plaquenil, antimalarial drug, 57
Pless, I. B., 139
Plienes, A. J., 160
Pollock, D. J., 82
Polyarticular JRA, 66
    application of ABA theory to, 66–67
    medical regimen of 14-year-old male
        with, 66
Pontious, S. L., 40
Pool, R., 155
Poppen, R. L., 64
Popper, K. R., 47
Portnoy, J. M., 2
Powell, C., 170
Powers, S. W., 159
Prednisone, corticosteroid, 57
Prescribed Intervals Method (PI), 105

Problems of adherence
    types/nature of, 70–71
Prochaska, J. O., 58, 59, 60, 61, 62
Prompting adherence, 129
    Hand-held PDA programs, 129
Psychometric standards of adherence
    clinical feasibility, utility, and relevance,
        111–112
    limiting "physiogenic bias," 110–111
Psychotherapeutic interventions, 138
Psychotherapy, 58, 59
Purviance, M. R., 64, 73

Q
Quittner, A. L., 7, 40, 50, 73, 79, 87, 88, 91,
        92, 93, 100, 102, 107, 123, 127,
        140, 141, 143, 160

R
Rabinovich, M., 6
Rachelefsky, G., 156
Radius, S. M., 10, 36, 37, 41, 42, 49
Raia, J., 35
Rai, S. N., 125
Rand, C., 95
Rand, C. S., 76, 79, 80, 83, 92, 93, 102
Rapoff, M. A., 4, 7, 8, 9, 27, 28, 36, 37, 40, 41,
        63, 64, 65, 69, 73, 77, 79, 84, 86,
        102, 117, 119, 121, 122, 130, 132,
        136, 138, 140, 142, 149, 151, 173,
        174, 177, 180, 182, 183, 184
Rashid, M., 23
Ratner, P., 155
Rayens, M. K., 153
RCTs, *see* Controlled clinical trials (RCTs)
Readability of written material
    formulas for calculating, 119*t*
    See also Educational strategies for
        improving adherence
Redding, C. A., 59
Reddington, C., 25, 34
Regimen-related correlates, 41–42
    adherence correlates to medical regimens,
        41–42
        costs, 41
        efficacy, 42
        side effects, 41–42
        type and complexity, 41
Reimers, S., 27
Reindenberg, B. E., 4
Remor, B., 13
Rescorla, L. A., 110
Research on pediatric medical adherence,
        ten ways to advance, 181–184

conduct multisite/randomized controlled
    intervention trials, 184
develop electronic monitor measures, 183
develop practical measures of disease
    activity and quality of life, 183
develop promotion strategies and ways
    to deliver interventions, 184
develop self-report measures, 182–183
develop standard scores/cut points for
    classifying people, 181
make theories relevant to pediatrics,
    181–182
prevention of anticipated declines over
    time, 183
settle on standard definition, 181
use of single-subject design
    methodology, 183
Reynolds, E., 170
Reynolds, L. A., 77
Richards, M. E., 40
Richardson, C., 165
Richardson, P., 163
Rieder, M. J., 42
Riegler, H. C., 63
Riekert, K., 92
Riekert, K. A., 79, 80
Riley, A. W., 107
Ritterband, L. M., 143
Roberts, C. M., 159
Roberts, G. M., 139
Roberts, M. C., 43, 119, 177, 180
Rock, D. L., 85
Rode, C. A., 107
Rodewald, L. E., 76
Rodrigues, A. F., 23
Rodriques, W. J., 6
Rohay, J., 153
Rosas, A., 37
Rosen, B., 148
Rosenbaum, P., 108
Rosenberg, A., 27
Rosen, C. S., 61
Rosen, D., 11
Rosenstock, I. M., 48, 50, 53
Rosenthal, R., 152
Ross, C. K., 27, 41
Roter, D. L., 177, 180
Roth, D. L., 61
Roth, H. P., 74, 82
Rounds, K. A., 151
Rowbothan, M. C., 113
Royle, M., 24
Rubin, D. H., 144, 156

Rubin, L. G., 42
Rubio, A., 82
Rudd, P., 76, 77, 81, 83, 84, 93, 102
Ruggiero, L., 59, 61, 62
Rule-governed behavior, 63
    problems/limitations, 64
Ryan, R. M., 65
Ryder, C., 92
Ryle, G., 116
Ryle, Gilbert (British philosopher), 116

S
Saadah, O. I., 23
Sahota, N., 152
Salazar, J. C., 170
Salomon, J., 13
Sanchez, J., 17
Santiago, J. V., 37, 40
Sanz, E. J., 2
Saputo, M., 150
Satin, W., 151
Schafer, L. C., 39, 41, 166
Schechter, K., 161
Scheier, L. M., 28
Schentag, J. J., 76, 77
Schlösser, M., 53
Schmidt, L. E., 17
Scholten, R. J., 157
Schwankovsky, L., 50
Schwartz-Lookinland, S., 150
Schwartz, R. H., 6
Schwarzer, R., 53
Schweitzer, J. B., 172
Scotti, J. R., 66
Screening
    process of, 69
    tool for adherence assessment, 69
SCT, *see* Social cognitive theory (SCT)
Sculerati, N., 6
Seale, J. P., 157
Secord, E., 171
Seid, M., 107
Seidman, L., 20
Selbmann, H., 4
Self-efficacy
    conceptual/methodological grounds,
        criticism on, 53
    enhancement, factors for, 55
    health-related behaviors, predictor
        of, 52, 53
    illness-specific scales for children/
        adolescents, 53
    influence on health, pathways, 52

Self-efficacy (*cont.*)
    judgments/outcome expectations, 52
    person–environment interactions,
        role in, 53
    sources, 52
    theory, 53 *f*
Self-management strategies, 138
    cognitive and contemporary
        behavior, 138
    problem-solving skills, 138
    psychotherapeutic interventions, 138
    treatments/diseases with positive/negative
        consequences, 139*t*
    See also Improvement strategies of
        adherence
Selimğlu, A., 20
Selimoglu, M. A., 24
Sergis-Davenport, E., 77, 170
Serrano-Ikkos, E., 31, 37, 38
SES, *see* Socioeconomic status (SES)
Sesselberg, T. S., 143
Shaw, J., 157
Sheeran, P., 57
Sheiner, L. B., 74
Shellmer, D. A., 83
Shemesh, E., 31, 38, 39, 40
Sherman, J. M., 94
Shingadia, D., 171
Siller, J., 37
Silverman, A. H., 166
Silverstein, J., 37, 77, 86
Simmons, F .E. R., 10
Simon, H. J., 92
Simon, P. M., 152
Simons, L. E., 50
Singer, J., 3
Singh, G., 107
Singh, J., 118, 119
Skinner, B. F., 63, 65, 66
Skyler, J. S., 37, 151
Slack, M. K., 40, 41, 42
SLE, *see* Systemic lupus
    erythematosus (SLE)
Sleasman, J. W., 25
Sly, R. M., 34
Smith, A. W., 36
Smith, C. F., 118, 119
Smith, M., 34
Smith, N. A., 157
Smith, S. D., 11, 37
Smith-Whitley, K., 29
Smyth, A., 144
Smyth, A. R., 94

Snodgrass, S. R., 38
Snyder, C. R., 8
Snyder, J., 167
Social cognitive theory (SCT)
    appraisal, 52–54
        self-efficacy theory, criticism, 53
    clinical implications, 54–55
        CF, strategies to adherence, 54
        clinicians, outcome expectancies, 55
        7-year-old female with CF, example, 54
    description, 51–52
        adherence tasks, challenges faced by
        children/adolescents, 52
        self-efficacy, pathways,
        see Self-efficacy
    proposed/promoted by Albert Bandura, 51
Socioeconomic status (SES), 37–38
Socolar, R., 135
Sokol, M. C., 35
Somerville, S. C., 36
Sood, M., 22
Spangler, D. L., 151
Spergel, J., 50
Spieth, L. E., 106, 107, 110
Sprague, J. R., 142
Srivastava, A., 24
Stack, C. M., 143
Standards, adherence
    accuracy, 103
    reliability, 103
        of interview/observational
        measures, 103
    validity, 103
Starfield, B., 107
Stark, L., 183, 184
Stark, L. J., 43, 151, 160, 169, 175
Starlight Foundation asthma program, "Quest
    for the Code," 144
Starr, M., 101
Steele, R. G., 30
Stein, R. E. K., 111
Stemmler, M. M., 41
Stern, R. S., 135
Stevens, B., 112
Stewart, S. M., 18, 37
Stiesmeyer, J., 156
Stinson, J. N., 112
Stoppelbein, L., 13
Storey, K., 142
Stork, P. P., 86
Strategies for assessment of adherence
    adherence measures, comparative
        performance, 94–102

assets/liabilities of adherence
measures, 74*t*
drug assays, 74–77
electronic monitors, 79–83
observation, 77–79
patient/parental reports, 86–94
pill counts, 83–84
provider estimates, 84–85
Stratman, A. C., 30
Strecher, V. J., 48, 50, 53
Strickland, D. E., 110
Stroebe, M. S., 50, 57
Stroebe, W., 50, 57
Strosahl, K. D., 66
Stuber, M., 34
Sturmey, P., 71, 72, 142
Swales, T., 89
Systemic lupus erythematosus (SLE), 57
medical regimen of 15-year-old female
with, 57
application of TRA/PB to, 58

T
Takiya, L., 177
Talpey, W. B., 5
Tamaroff, M. H., 10, 39, 49
Taplin, S. H., 55
Target behaviors for assessing adherence,
selection of
guidelines
baseline all behaviors, 71–72
critical or "keystone" behaviors, 72
easy to change behaviors, 73
problematic or disturbing behaviors, 72
Taylor, W. R., 34
Tebbi, C. K., 7, 11, 37, 38, 40
Technology-based interventions, 143–145
See also Improvement strategies
of adherence
Templin, T. N., 44
Tepper, V., 90
Tepper, V. J., 25
Terdal, L. G., 69, 71, 78, 79
Theories
ABA theory, 63–67
clinicians, reasons for acceptance of, 47
definition, 47
HBM, 48–51
researchers, impact on, 47
SCT, 51–55
TRA/PB, 55–58
TTM, 58–62
See also individual

Theory of reasoned action/planned behaviour
(TRA/PB), 56 *f*
appraisal, 57
clinical implications, 57–58
SLE, strategies to adherence, 58
15-year-old female with SLE,
example, 57
description, 55–56
attitude, prediction of behavioral
outcomes, 55–56
behavioral intentions, factors, 56
Theory of Reasoned Action (TRA), 55
Therapeutic Coverage (TC), 105
Thomas, A. M., 89, 138
Thomas, J., 86
Thompson, R. E., 23, 96
Thompson, R. H., 159
Time-out handout, 136 *f* –137 *f*
See also Educational strategies for
improving adherence
Tinkelman, D. G., 10, 151, 157
Todd, J. T., 65, 66
Toll, D., 125
Tommasini, A., 24
Topolski, T. D., 107
Tor, M., 94
Tourangeau, R., 93
Transplant failures
lower adherence to immunosuppressive
drugs, 33
Transtheoretical model (TTM)
appraisal, 59–61
TTM stages, criticism, 61
behavioral processes of change, types
cognitive/self-mediated thought
processes, 67
environmental contingencies, 67
behavioral stages of change
action, 59
contemplation, 59
maintenance, 59
precontemplation, 59
preparation, 59
clinical implications, 61–62
Type 1 diabetes, strategies
to adherence, 62
16-year-old male with Type 1 diabetes,
example, 61–62
description, 58–59
decisional balance/self-efficacy, 59
systems of psychotherapy, applied
to, 59
"transtheoretical," origin of term, 59

Transtheoretical model (TTM) (*cont.*)
dimensions of, 60*t*
processes of change, 59
health-related behaviors, 59
TRA/PB, *see* Theory of reasoned
action/planned behaviour
(TRA/PB)
Triadic reciprocal causation model, *see* Social
cognitive theory (SCT)
Trueworthy, R. C., 11
Tuberculosis, reemergence
adherence failures, effects, 34
Tucker, C. M., 31, 38, 40, 91
Türkan, Y., 20
Turk, D. C., 65
Type 1 diabetes, 61–62
medical regimen of 16-year-old male with,
61–62
application of TTM to, 62

U
Urquhart, J., 3, 35, 79, 80, 82

V
Valenzuela, D., 86
Vandereycken, W., 3
Vanderpool, G. E., 151
Van Dyke, R. B., 25, 41, 90
Van Es, S. M., 40, 42, 157
Van Slyke, D. A., 135
Varasteh, L. T., 8
Variables that predict adherence
cues to action, 48
to medical regimens
clinicians, role of, 67
perceived barriers/ benefits, 48
perceived severity/susceptibility, 48
Varni, J. W., 65, 77, 107, 112, 169, 170
Vedanarayanan, V. V., 38
Verbally controlled (rule-governed) behavior,
see Self-efficacy
Verbal persuasion
'pep talks,' 55
Verbrugge, R. R., 35
Vrijens, B., 36

W
Wadsworth, L. D., 20
Wagner, D. J., 35
Wagner, E. H., 36
Walco, G. A., 39
Walders, N., 9, 10, 37, 79
Walker, L. S., 135
Wallander, J. L., 43, 65

Ware, J. E., 107
Warzak, W. J., 142
Watrous, M., 107
Webb, T. L., 57
Weber, E., 79
Wehlou, K., 42
Weintraub, M., 82
Weizman, Z., 19
Wells, J. A., 110
Wentzell, K. J., 164
Werner, R. J., 5, 7
Westman, E., 24
White-coat compliance, 3
Whitehead, B., 31
Wicker, A. W., 47
Wiebe, D. J., 18, 40
Wiener, L., 92
Wildman, B. G., 78, 79, 102
Williams, P. L., 25, 39
Williams, R., 150
Williams, S. L., 105
Willies-Jacobo, L. J., 37
Wilson, D. B., 152
Wilson, D. P., 18
Wilson, K. G., 53, 54, 66
Wilson, N. W., 37
Wing, R. R., 18, 19, 77
Winnick, S., 125
Winter, M. E., 74, 75, 76, 77
Wise, R. A., 76, 83, 93, 102
Wishner, W. J., 1
Wolf, F. M., 181
Wood, L. V., 92
Wood, P. R., 10
Wood, S. F., 42
Wu, Y. P., 119, 177, 180
Wyatt, R. A., 9
Wynn, K. S., 39
Wyplj, D., 36
Wysocki, T., 39, 43, 89, 151, 152, 167, 168

Y
Yachha, S. K., 24
Yaffe, S. J., 4
Yamada, J., 112
Yang, M. C. K., 143
Yao, X., 177
Yoman, J., 64, 142

Z
Zacharin, M., 23
Zaleski, S., 118
Zeevi, N., 19
Zeiger, R., 50

Zelikovsky, N., 50, 83
Zeltzer, L. K., 155
Zevon, M. A., 40
Zhang, M., 153
Zifferblatt, S. M., 63

"Ziggy Theorem," 106
Zigo, M. A., 151
Ziman, R., 9
Zora, J. A., 10
Zunzunegui, M. V., 26

Breinigsville, PA USA
10 June 2010
239595BV00001B/19/P